The Colour of Sex

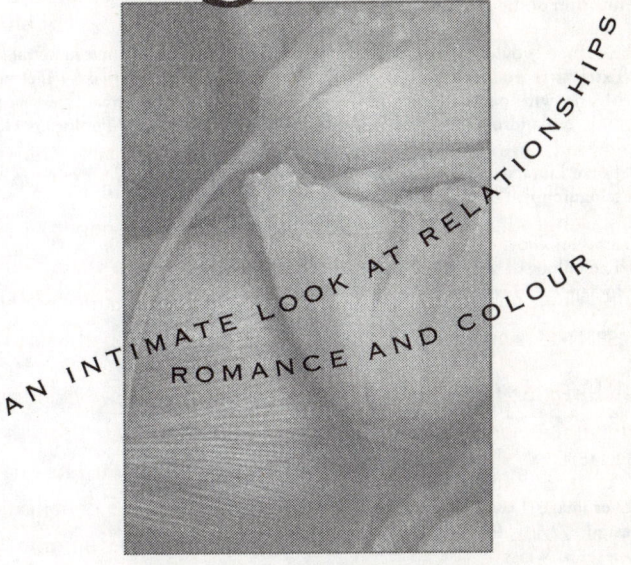

AN INTIMATE LOOK AT RELATIONSHIPS
ROMANCE AND COLOUR

**Lynn Champion
Judy Scott-Kemmis**

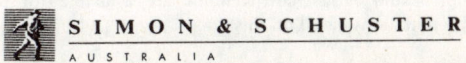

THE COLOUR OF SEX

First published in Australia in 1999 by
Simon & Schuster (Australia) Pty Limited
20 Barcoo Street, East Roseville NSW 2069

Reprinted 1999

A Viacom Company
Sydney New York London Toronto Tokyo Singapore

© Lynn Champion and Judy Scott-Kemmis 1999

All rights reserved. No part of this publication may be reproduced, stored in a retrieval system, or transmitted, in any form or by any means, electronic, mechanical, photocopying, recording or otherwise, without the prior permission of the publisher in writing.

The authors would like to thank the following for the use of their material:
Extracts reproduced from *The Naked Ape* and *The Human Animal* by Desmond Morris, with permission of BBC Worldwide Limited; *Nonverbal Communication* by L. Malandro and L. Barker, Addison Wesley Educational Publishers USA.

National Library of Australia
Cataloguing-in-Publication data

Champion, Judy.
 The colour of sex : an intimate look at relationships, romance and colour.

 ISBN 0 7318 0821 5.

 1. Color – Psychological aspects. 2. Color – Therapeutic use. 3. Sex. I. Scott-Kemmis, Judy. II. Title.

152.145

Cover image: David Wasserman
Design: DiZign Pty Ltd
Typeset in Weiss
Printed in Australia by Australian Print Group

Lynn Champion and Judy Scott-Kemmis would like to hear your comments about *The Colour of Sex*. If you are interested in receiving information on a future newsletter, workshops and other activities, please write enclosing a self addressed, stamped envelope to:

IN LIVING COLOUR
PO Box 31
Balmain 2041
Australia

Lynn Champion and Judy Scott-Kemmis are available for seminars and conference presentations based on this book.

Contents

PREFACE   VI

SECTION ONE:
absolutely fabulous Colours

CHAPTER 1   2
colourful relationships
... colour, sex, and you
What is colour? Colour quiz.

SECTION TWO
romancing

CHAPTER 2   8
the seducer's notebook
... colour, sex, romance and you

Nine steps to seduction; How sensual are you?; How sexual are you?; Your courting style; What colours should you wear?; Where to on the first date?

CHAPTER 3   37
romancing the body
... colour, sex, clothes and you

Outerwear; Underwear; The colour and sensuality quotient; Nightwear.

CHAPTER 4   58
the biology of sex
... colourful body, colourful seduction

Visual appearance; The sound of the voice and the choice of language; Scent signalling; Smooth skin; Touching behaviour; The colour and biology of sex.

SECTION THREE
bedroom behaviours

CHAPTER 5   76
up close and colourful
... colour in the bedroom

Identifying your overall colour scheme; Colour psychology; Creating balance with colour; Creating your own oasis.

CHAPTER 6
intimate design
... how bedroom style plays its part

101

A bedroom questionnaire;
What your answers reveal;
Nine readily identifiable styles of
intimate design.

CHAPTER 7
master strokes
... significant simplicities for success

142

Clear away the clutter; Begin the creative
make-over of your bedroom; Change the
way you do things; Remedies for the bedroom;
What to wear to bed;
Romancing and seducing each style;
Afterplay.

SECTION FOUR
living the Sensual and romantic life

CHAPTER 8
the golden rules
... creating loving, intimate relationships

176

Preface

Sex is a fascinating topic, happy relationships always the desired state, and loving romance a top scorer on most people's wish list. Tie those together with colour, and practical suggestions for harmony, and we know lives will change.

Our research has enabled us to reassess romantic and sexual behaviours and link them with colour choices in a practical way. As researchers and workshop presenters we have been fascinated by communication, image and colour psychology for nearly 20 years. One evening at a marketing seminar we realised it was time to explain to others our ideas, knowledge and experience with colour psychology so they could live the strategies we had understood for so long. We decided to start with sex and colour, knowing the book would not be about explicit sexual behaviours, rather about sensuality and improving sex by improving communication.

In *The Colour of Sex* we explore the well-researched patterns of colour choices. Throughout, we explain the emotional and physical meaning of colours and place them in a practical context for you. We have information to help you read your partner's sexual and romantic moods without you saying a word, to understand the subconscious message in every bedroom (colour and style choices do that), to know the nine steps to seduction with a new partner and to provide you with remedies for better relationships and romance. And lots more. We found the entire project fascinating, filled with waves of insight and awakenings. Certainly there were times when both of us found the research and writing absolutely seductive. Imagine how you would feel sitting at a table covered with an array of underwear, and handling each example to assess the colour and sensuality quotient – or as we refer to it, CSQ. (See Chapter 4 'Romancing the Body').

Our background and experience have helped shape this book. We have both lived the highs and lows – both of us have been married, raised children, divorced and subsequently been involved in loving relationships. We have not only used our own experiences; we have interviewed many colleagues and professional communicators to gain insights into how to enhance romance, love and relationships. And at the same time, we researched and tested colour theories as well.

Our businesses for many years have concentrated on just these factors too. Lynn Champion is a business speaker, winner of colour and image awards in Australia and the USA, a former Australian Executive Woman of the Year, and media broadcaster on communication and image topics. She majored in anthropology at the University of Sydney. It is her interest in anthropology, social behaviours and verbal and non-verbal communication which she has used to contribute to this book.

Judy Scott-Kemmis, a graduate of the School of Colour and Design is a well-known colour expert. Her work involves analysing and interpreting colour usage in all its applications for home and business, as well as designing and decorating artwork for manufactured products. She brings years of colour knowledge and research to this book. Currently studying sociology and psychology at the Southern Cross University, Lismore, Judy's passion is the impact and effect of colour on our psyches.

The Colour of Sex. It is fun, frank and filled with simple truths. It leads you gently to happy relationships, enhanced romance and sex. It is for all of you who are beginning a new relationship and for all of you in established partnerships. It changes lives.

Lynn Champion

Judy Scott-Kemmis

SECTION
one

absolutely fabulous Colours

Colour is pervasive. It enriches emotions, relationships and lives.

CHAPTER 1

colourful relationships

... colour,
sex,
and you

Weave the threads of sensuality and colour powerfully into your life. Colour is a fabulous way to enhance romance, love and relationships. Team information on sensual colour psychology with positive communication strategies and notice the changes in your relationship. Colourful changes. You will enjoy them, absolutely. *The Colour of Sex* provides you with romantic remedies for tired relationships, romantic concepts to make a first date lead to a lasting relationship, (if that's what you want) and fascinating ideas to take you to loving seduction. It is for lovers, spouses and new partners.

We have combined knowledge of the effects of colour with powerful information on human behaviours, sensuality and relationships. Much of the information is new. What is not new is sex drive. Perhaps happy sex has been put on the back burner for you because of stress or circumstances you can't change. Nevertheless, if you are single, you are still driven to look for a partner, enjoy the romance of a new relationship, lust after the sex and sensuality which go hand in hand with it, and set in place commitment and behaviours to establish a long-lasting loving relationship. And you are not alone. Men and women in long-term relationships yearn for all the substance of sexual success as well as romance. For a variety of reasons the loving seems to get buried in comfortable practical security.

What is colour?

The simplest definition is that colour is the vibration of light energy. It has been proven over many years that colour affects emotions, moods, health, wellbeing, spiritual awareness and the mind at conscious and subconscious levels. A series of grey overcast days subdues the spirit of most people. When sunshine and blue skies appear again, spirits lift. Walking into a yellow painted room gives a sense of brightness and warmth. A stroll in a park where there are plenty of green trees brings a sense of well-being and harmony.

COLOUR AFFECTS EMOTIONS, MOODS, HEALTH, WELLBEING, SPIRITUAL AWARENESS AND THE MIND AT CONSCIOUS AND SUBCONSCIOUS LEVELS

Colour influences desire, sensuality and sex. Colour isn't the only factor which will build a romance to a sexual outcome, but understanding which colours stimulate desire and which don't will give you knowledge and power. You probably take for granted the myriad of colours around you each day without appreciating their presence and their effect. How often have you looked into the centre of a flower and noticed the variety of colours there, or taken note of the many unusual colours in your partner's eyes, or the subtle tones in your own skin colouring? Pause for a moment and notice the natural variations in colour. Try to imagine a world without colour. How would you feel if everything was only black and white?

Colour blind? Perhaps you think colour information does not apply to you. However, as colour is simply the vibration of light energy, it affects us whether we can see it or not. Visually impaired people understand this and many can 'feel' colours very accurately. None of us see colour in exactly the same way or to the same degree of intensity, yet it still affects each of us on a subconscious level.

As we begin the journey with you, have courage. A new level of intimacy awaits you. Are you open to discovering and reaping the benefits of a conscious use of colour in close personal relationships? Is a new level of commitment and caring in your relationship important to your wellbeing and happiness? We are sure you have answered yes. Congratulations. You are ready to take the colour plunge. Colour is pervasive. It enriches emotions, relationships and lives.

A NEW LEVEL OF INTIMACY AWAITS YOU

COLOUR ENRICHES EMOTIONS, RELATIONSHIPS AND LIVES

Colour Quiz

To get you started on the tapestry of colour and rich relationships answer the Colour Quiz questions. Choose the colour which you think best answers the following questions:

1. For seductive underwear, what do you dare wear:
   GREEN   BLUE   RED   PURPLE?

2. Mystery and control? Would you wear:
   RED   WHITE   YELLOW   BLACK?

3. Which colour for social chat:
   RED   ORANGE   WHITE   BLACK?

4. Bedroom times – do you love to criticise? Which colour do you avoid so you can harmonise:
   RED   ORANGE   WHITE   YELLOW?

5. New ideas, experimentation – which colour will give you inspiration:
   YELLOW   SILVER   BLACK   BLUE?

6. Burning the candle at both ends? Which colour will make amends:
   BLUE   VIOLET   GREEN   RED?

7. New beginnings, a fresh start, which colour to capture your heart:
   WHITE   RED   GREEN   ORANGE?

8. Imagination, inspiration, which colour is artistically creative:
   BLUE   WHITE   PURPLE   RED?

9. For peace, calm and order, which colour reduces stress
   ORANGE   RED   BLUE   BROWN?

Answers:
1: *red;* 2: *black;* 3: *orange;* 4: *yellow;* 5: *yellow;* 6: *green;*
7: *white;* 8: *purple;* 9: *blue.*

Soon you will understand why these answers are true.

Be seduced by colour and communication concepts.

SECTION two

romancing

Seduction
is best
sipped and
savoured
slowly.

CHAPTER 2

the seducer's notebook

... colour, sex, romance and you

Ah, the excitement of the romantic chase. The fantasies, the lust, the yearnings and heightened insecurities. Your body becomes more sensitive to sounds, smells and certainly to touch. You see the object of your interest through not only rose coloured glasses but also through a gold tinged magnifying glass. You remember what all of this is like don't you? One of life's most exciting experiences has overtaken you.

Romance takes careful consideration. Nevertheless when you meet someone appealing, you are tempted to proceed because someone has stirred your senses and emotions. A new relationship may be about to begin. All the emotional and physical signs are seemingly present: the longer-than-average eye contact, the flirtatious smiles, the appreciation of the love interest's face or body, the sensual bantering which goes on between you, or simply the chemistry telling you 'yes'. This time you may well want to achieve a 'fine romance' and not just 'another romance'. So let's look at the areas you need to consider:

- What are the steps to seduction?
- How sensual are you?
- How sexual are you?
- What is your romancing style?
- What colours should you wear early in the relationship?
- Where to on the first date?

Nine steps to seduction

You see someone who appeals to you. You eye one another from a distance and contemplate the first move. The sequence for seduction in all cultures is nearly always the same, give or take a few details, advises Desmond Morris in his television series and book, *The Human Animal*.

THE SEQUENCE FOR SEDUCTION IN ALL CULTURES IS NEARLY ALWAYS THE SAME

1. We softly smile and with a slightly longer than average eye contact, we signal our sexual interest.

2. If the soft smile is returned, we make voice contact. Trivial conversation is begun and then some background information collected. 'What type of work do you do?' 'Have you worked there long?' ' Do you know the host well?' 'What are your hobbies?' 'Are you married?'

While talking, we check the manner and style of speaking and if we don't like what we hear we end the relationship then and there.

3. We prolong the eye gaze and can notice the pupil dilation. The pupils cannot lie if you are in natural sheltered lighting. If there is interest, the pupils enlarge and seem very black. Uninterested? You will notice pin spot pupils. If that is the case, you might as well give up unless you know the small pupils are the result of medication, drugs or an extra abundance of light in the setting.

4. Physical contact is the next step in this accepted sequence. Just the lightest touch of his clothing by a woman when she comments on the tie, jacket or whatever she admires, or the picking off of lint from his shoulder. For him, he may hold

her hand to assist, or guide her through a doorway by lightly placing his hand on the small of her back.

5. Closer contact can be introduced by the arm around the shoulder, holding hands, walking arm in arm or stroking the upper arm area once the couple discovers they like to be with each other. Sometimes step 7 comes into this section.

6. The full embrace comes next, often accompanied by mouth to mouth kissing.

7. Hand to head is the next phase. This is a special sense of intimacy because the head is a strongly guarded region of the body. So to let someone caress your face, or touch your hair transmits the signal of openness and vulnerability. To initiate the touching is your way of testing the water. We only let friends caress our hair and face. These are seemingly safe, but very intimate actions.

8. The hands of the companion are permitted to stray over the body. The first touch may be a stroking of the knee if the couple is seated, and stroking of the shoulder, if standing. If these relatively safe and curved areas on both men and women are accepted, then the relationship will be tested further. Signals of serious sexual contact have begun. When hands start to caress the more intimate regions of the partner's body all pretence has to cease. This is the time to encourage or discourage. It is up to you.

It may take a long time to reach step 8. It may happen reasonably quickly. Only you two can decide. Consider lingering longer over some of the steps to give you both an opportunity to enjoy and understand each other. Any one who moves too quickly will find themselves in trouble. Now you know why the fool at the staff party who moves to step 8 before going through all the previous steps will inevitably be rejected.

9. The next phase is full sexual intimacy, involving hand to breast or chest, mouth to nipple, hand to bottom, hand to genitals and finally genitals to genitals. You have been seduced. You have seduced. And you approved every step along the way. Whether you give approval of the sexual act itself, later, is a different matter.

The sequence as outlined has to happen. Occasionally a couple will slightly alter the order. Perhaps with your last lover you brought in for example, step 7, hand to head, earlier. Doing this doesn't mean you leave out the other steps – you will reinforce them with your other behaviours. Arriving at step 9 will not occur without the approval of many aspects of communication. Seduction after all is not just a physical process. The conversations, the ideas, the behaviours and the personality of the potential lover are all part of the equation. Either party has the right to stop the sequence at any stage. If a woman allows a man to arrive at step 9 and then says 'stop' when the green lights have been showing in stages 1 to 8, she is accused very roundly of being 'a tease'. Yet sometimes, all the touching in steps 8 and 9 can be frightening and anxiety-producing, so both men and women may choose to slow down the process considerably.

SEDUCTION IS NOT JUST A PHYSICAL PROCESS

Not all sexual encounters are designed for slow enduring romance and long-term relationships. Some people want a one-night stand. For whatever reasons, a passionate encounter is

Romancing

their focus. There is no time, nor the inclination, to create a long-lasting relationship. The process in this case will be well and truly accelerated. In any case steps 1 to 7 must happen for both partners to feel involved and not feel taken for granted.

All humans want closeness and a special companion. Ultimately the passionate, quick fling approach to romance and sex is unsatisfactory. If you've had enough of that lifestyle, the time has come to slow down the steps to seduction, enjoy the view and feelings along the way and take time to discover and enjoy the new person in your life.

TAKE YOUR TIME

SEDUCTION IS BEST SIPPED AND SAVOURED SLOWLY

The nine-step sequence of seduction applies to well-established relationships as well as new ones. Romance for even long-term lovers needs the nine steps to ensure the most intimate and loving atmosphere in the home and bedroom. The fact that you know each other very well is no reason to skip a step or two. Take your time. Enjoy the steps. They place you both on the path to sexual happiness and fulfilment. Most of the steps for long-term partners could be called foreplay, to be enjoyed at any time of the day, some in the morning perhaps and continued in the evening. Seduction is best sipped and savoured slowly.

How sensual are you?

Some of you have no difficulty answering 'very'. Others are more moderate in their acknowledgment. Some may be saying 'not very'. Sensuality has a strong bearing on romance. The more sensual you are the more chance the relationship has to grow into a 'fine romance'. 'Sensual' as defined by the *Oxford*

Dictionary means 'of or depending on the senses only and not the intellect or spirit'. You know the five senses well: sight, touch, sound, taste and smell. Add the sixth sense, intuition, as an important ingredient for relationships too.

A sensual person is not only aware of the senses, but uses them every day to build intimacy and communication. Sensuality is often heightened during the early days of the romance. It's obvious in the preening you go through to *look* just right. Your body language supports it as well. You will tend to lean forward, make strong eye contact and have the repertoire of invitational signals when you flirt. You may run a hand through your hair, turn to be full frontal to the new love interest and smile frequently. These are all powerful visual clues for sensuality.

> **ADD THE SIXTH SENSE, INTUITION, AS AN IMPORTANT INGREDIENT FOR RELATIONSHIPS TOO**

You need your home to look attractive too so you feel proud when your guest comes calling. Can't afford the home decor you yearn for? Choose some splashes of happy colours as accents in the meantime. Something as simple as a vase of flowers or new and colourful cushions, will make you look and feel confident. Having a completely bland colour scheme doesn't send a sensual message about you.

Keep your home clean and tidy. Nothing turns off a potential partner faster than messiness, so get rid of clutter and dirt. This will give you a great sense of freedom and clarity as though a load has been lifted. The truth is, it has. Clean it up, brighten it up and watch your spirits and confidence soar.

Your sensuality is also obvious in the *touching* behaviour you show your new partner. Follow the normal rules of touching safe areas of the body such as arms, hands, elbows and shoulders. Perhaps touching is difficult for you. Have courage. Most men and women don't get enough touching in their adult life, although we all need it. The touching behaviour which works best is the light touch. Don't grab. Don't linger, until you really wish to hold hands across the table.

THE TOUCHING BEHAVIOUR WHICH WORKS BEST IS THE LIGHT TOUCH

Touching is a sign of approval, acceptance and closeness. The light touch also tells others who may be interested in your new friend to stay away. It telegraphs ownership. Don't allow your hands to stray near intimate areas on your friend's body until you are sure you're invited there.

Does your partner enjoy being massaged around the neck and shoulders? This is a friendly and caring action after a tiring day at work. As your romance develops, become good at giving a body massage with the best smelling oils (men like pine and other refreshing oils rather than the sweet ones preferred by women), soft towels, a warm room and with pleasant music in the background. Insist on your massage too.

And men, please remember to shave. There is nothing more annoying for a woman, or less pleasing, than having her chin and jaw rubbed sore by stubble as you kiss her.

Develop your tactile ability and identify the feelings of touch you enjoy most. Touch surfaces, fabrics and furniture, not only people. After you have cleaned your home for your guest, touch ornaments, touch furniture surfaces, feel your towels and feel your sheets and pillow cases. Derive pleasure from feeling the differences. Which ones appeal? Run your hands over surfaces and objects. Enjoy the variety of warmth and cool as well as hard, soft, slippery, smooth, and textured.

Your sensuality is also obvious in the *voice* you use and what you say. At the beginning of relationships the sound of laughter and a certain tone of voice telegraph interest. The tone to intrigue is warm and if possible deep, both on the phone and in person. In general, men and women respond more positively to deeper rather than higher pitched voices.

Some potential partners don't say much. Others are very talkative. Whatever your style, don't talk a lot about very personal matters early on. Remain a little mysterious. This is sure to intrigue your friend. Leave him or her wanting to know more. Women are most likely to spill the beans on childhood, previous relationships, details of how they got on well with their fathers but not their mothers, etc. within the first hour of meeting someone.

Stop it. Ask questions. Allow silences. It gives the pleasure of quiet times. Overcome the desire to fill silences. Let them be. Nobody wants to be on the receiving end of a barrage of information. While you are so busy talking you're not listening.

To enhance the sense of hearing, think about all the sounds that give you pleasure. Then discover the sounds your partner enjoys. Does he or she like the quiet sound of the country and the beach, or the excitement of cafés in the city? Getting on well with others is a matter of understanding their likes and dislikes. Does your friend like classical music, country music, hard rock, opera? Or perhaps he or she prefers to

> **TO ENHANCE THE SENSE OF HEARING, THINK ABOUT ALL THE SOUNDS THAT GIVE YOU PLEASURE**

whistle or sing. Keep a note and do something about it when you entertain or give gifts. Music should be a background player to the most important event: your relationship.

Your sensuality can be expressed in the *taste* of the food you serve and the food you choose to eat when you are with your new love. Only serve the freshest food when your new friend comes for a meal. You don't have to buy the most expensive, merely good quality. This is not the time for tired leftovers, dubious snacks or fatty takeaways. Your choice of coffee, tea, soft drinks or alcohol, as well as their presentation, speaks volumes about how you value yourself and your friend. A glass of water served with a lemon slice in an attractive glass has more style than a sugary soft drink.

Food is not only a source of pleasure, it is a comfort too. It fills in the spaces in your relationship, gives you good topics to discuss and pleasures to enjoy. The visual presentation of the food you give your friend is linked to the taste. Go the extra mile to make the entire eating experience of even the simplest snack attractive. Take time to colour coordinate the plates, napkins, cups etc. and to be a good host.

The *smell* of your home, your kitchen, your bathroom and eventually your bedroom are indicators of your sensuality as well. Clean, fresh and natural smells are enticing. Air your home regularly. Having a fragrant home is appealing and you may decide to use pot-pourri or oil burners using essential oils throughout your home. If you do, choose just one key fragrance at a time so you don't confuse the senses. Florals in summer and spring and something more aromatic or

CLEAN, FRESH AND NATURAL SMELLS ARE ENTICING

spicy for autumn and winter is a good way to go. Fresh flowers with an attractive perfume are always a winner as well. According to Feng Shui, fragrance in a home creates good *chi* or energy.

When it comes to wearing perfume or aftershave, less is more. You don't have to wear fragrance at all if that is your style. When you want to, do some research. A fragrance to complement you is worth seeking. Discover what works best on you. Is it oriental, floral, woody, fresh, classic or a mix of two of these? Spend some time at the fragrance counters of department stores and explain your personality and interests. A good fragrance consultant, by looking at your colouring and listening to your story will be able to suggest a few perfumes or aftershaves. Try a maximum of two on your wrists that day. Sniff them for the next few hours to decide how you feel about them and how they blend with your skin chemistry. If one of them doesn't sing to you, go back another day and try two more. Keep going until you find a fragrance which makes you feel sensual. Many people have two favourites, one for day and a heavier one for evening. Or one for summer and one for winter.

LET THE FRAGRANCE BE INTIMATE WITH YOU

When you apply your favourite, be discreet. That's the secret. Let the fragrance be intimate with you. For women it's best to put it on your skin under your clothes. Not on your neck and wrists, where its scent can overpower. Men using aftershave should just lightly, lightly, lightly, splash it on the face. The message for both men and women? Just because you can't smell it yourself after ten minutes is no reason to reapply. Resist. Others know you have it on. Women often feel more sensual and responsive when they smell men's fragrances. It must be subtle so it draws you in and leaves you wanting more.

Take a new look at yourself. Decide to involve the senses as much as possible in your life. Be as sensual as you can. Examine what you do each day to recognise and gratify your sensuality. Then you can bring that awareness to your romance. What can you do from tonight to make yourself more in tune with your senses of sight, touch, sound, taste and smell?

BE AS SENSUAL AS YOU CAN

It's not only becoming more aware, it's translating it into action in your relationship. For a successful relationship and added romance, choose positive action for all the senses:

1. present the best visual appearance of yourself
2. give attention to your grooming
3. have the best communication possible
4. make every room in your home attractive
5. have the best and cleanest smells in your home
6. have the most pleasant musical sounds in your home
7. tidy your garden, your yard and your car
8. have the best tastes in food without worrying about being an expert chef
9. have the courage to lightly touch a friend, to reach out and show emotion without anyone feeling overwhelmed

Challenge yourself to work on these areas. You know deep down the areas you are sloppy in. They're ones you don't feel very confident about too. Do something about them. You won't become a fabulous and sensual person overnight. You will however become a confidently sensual person who is not afraid to express your desires.

How sexual are you?

Now this is a loaded question. Perhaps it is time to look at your previous sexual history and behaviour so you can be better prepared for bed in this new relationship. And now, the million dollar question: what is your objective, your purpose, your aim with your new partner? If it is merely to have sex, you won't want to be reading any further. Just do it in the tried and true manner you have succeeded with in the past. If, however, you want an intimate, loving and long-lasting romantic relationship stay with us.

This book is about long-term happy times and good sex. We are not about to give explicit sexual encouragement. Rather we want you to consider:

- are you impatient as a lover? Once aroused do you get the two of you into bed quickly? Then after a little foreplay (five minutes maximum) move towards intercourse?
- are you a patient lover? Perhaps you have worked out the short- and long-term benefits of patience. When you slow down the process of foreplay, often beginning hours before undressing with light touching, smiles, banter and kissing, you build anticipation. Women love it. Men adore it.
- do you have patience with sensual undressing and with foreplay in bed?
- do you experiment with a few positions when you are having sex?
- do you ask your partner what he or she would like and insist on an answer?
- do you check on other days in quiet conversation if there are some other things you can do to enhance the sexual encounters?

- do you mix a good quota of sensuality with your sexuality?
- is your aim to give pleasure to your partner as well as being personally satisfied?
- do you dress to seduce?
- do you consider the very important visual aspects of seduction including clothing, bedroom appearance, lighting and bedding?

When you take a good look at your sexual behaviour you learn about yourself. Have you been really happy with the sex you've had in the past? What's been missing? Your style in bed reflects your personality and behaviour style out of bed. Change one and you change the other. You can't blame your partner forever.

HAVE YOU BEEN REALLY HAPPY WITH THE SEX YOU'VE HAD IN THE PAST?

Fast movers, fast talkers, fast decision makers are generally fast lovers. Creative thinkers are generally creative lovers. Slow talkers, movers and decision makers are generally slower lovers. And remember, they always say 'watch the quiet ones'.

Who's to say you can't mix these? Variety, and stretching your comfort zone around sexual behaviour is good for you and your romance.

Being more proactive in your job, your home, your life and now your love life will really pay off. It is the key. Do a little day-dreaming about some wonderful sensual experiences. Good sex begins with good sensuality.

What do you really want in your sexual experience? More variety for you in bed? Give more variety. More passion from a partner? Be more passionate. More time spent in foreplay? Work out a way you can do it. Offer to massage your partner or have a bubble bath or dress in sexy clothes. In other words, be proactive instead of reactive. And later, much later, not in bed, tell your partner what you really like.

GOOD SEX BEGINS WITH GOOD SENSUALITY

It's up to you to teach people how to treat you. It's never too late to start.

What is your communication style during a relationship?

How you communicate with a sexual partner mirrors how you communicate everyday with the world.

Here is a significant question for you: what are you doing and how are you doing it, when you know you are at your very best in a communication situation? What we mean by this is: there are times in our lives and relationships when we have an entranced audience (of one or more than one) and we feel so powerful, so in charge, so the centre of rapt attention. We are speaking and behaving in a way that feels so good, sounds so right and looks so accomplished. It may happen to you only occasionally. It may happen to you frequently. Think it through. Once you have identified the way you communicate when you are in this type of situation, you may decide that's what you always want to be like. You may well wonder why you change this best style for you for more submissive or more aggressive behaviours sometimes. Look at the reasons.

Your courting style

'Courting' is a word we don't use much these days. Courting is the first step in the intricate process of intimate relationship building. It means 'to pay court to; make love to; to entice' according to the *Oxford Dictionary*. To be courtly means 'being polished and refined in manners'. So your courting style means the manners and refinements you use with a potential partner to favourably impress, romance and entice.

To fully understand your courting style when you are with a person who captivates you, sit down, a piece of note-paper and a pen handy and write the strategies, the enticements and the romantic behaviours you have used with former partners. You know in your heart the ones which work for you.

As a man, do you let women chase you, cook for you early in the relationship, take you out for dinner, phone you often or are you more the traditional Romeo who protects and courteously opens doors and knows he wants do the chasing?

As a woman, are you mysteriously unavailable and keep a man guessing or are you openly sensual, flirtatious and talkative about your needs and desires? There are hundreds of courting behaviours. Look closely at your own. You can separate them from normal behaviour by recognising the special things you do. There is no right or wrong courting behaviour. Our purpose in asking you to list yours, whether you are in a relationship or not, is to give you personal insight. Your flirting/courting behaviours will be the ones you resort to again and again in all relationships. They are your guidelines for getting on with partners and potential partners. You probably learned them long ago and think you have perfected them. In a long-term relationship, look with fresh eyes at the behaviours you used to seduce your partner some time back, and reinvent them.

Elizabeth's list

We asked Elizabeth, who is in her late 40s, to list her courting behaviours when she went out on a first date and after much honest consideration and embarrassment about her modus operandi, this is the list she came up with:

1. When I like someone, early on in the relationship I touch his hands, or arm or sometimes even his face easily. Being very honest with myself, it's because I know that touching begins the bonding process. Being more honest, I know I need to be touched too. So touching him satisfies some of my needs.
2. I am talkative and am prepared to reveal intimate details (not sexual but personal) about my life.
3. I am good at getting a man to talk about himself. He will often say at the end of a dinner date, 'I don't usually talk about myself so much'.
4. I make good eye contact and smile a lot.
5. I laugh at his jokes and encourage him to tell me more. In fact, I make him the key player.
6. I allow him to open doors for me, pull out my chair and make decisions about wine.
7. I wear a subtle perfume.
8. I wear an attractive outfit that is stylish and not too sexy.
9. Unless it is a very casual date, I wear high heels.
10. I wear sexy underwear so I feel good, although there is no way he is going to see them on the first date.
11. I show some leg.
12. My make-up is carefully applied and my hair well groomed.
13. I sit opposite him so his focus of attention is on me.
14. As we walk from the restaurant, if I like him, I let my arm brush his.

15. If I like him, I kiss him on the cheek as I thank him for the evening.

16. When I speak to him next on the phone I thank him once more for the pleasant time we had.

17. In person or on the phone, I always make him laugh, not uproariously, more because I say unusual things.

18. I become very personal on the telephone. I want to break down any formality and allow us to move on with shared special times.

19. My home is always very neat and tidy with lovely flowers near the entrance.

20. My bedroom always looks good and has a sense of romance in it. This is not for him at this stage, but for me. It makes me feel romantically confident.

Elizabeth has had some very successful relationships and some not so good. She has made a conscious decision now to be less proactive and let a man do the hunting and chasing. Being more mysterious and revealing less about herself early on will be her new modus operandi. She realises she has told some new men almost everything very early in the relationship. She admits when she doesn't hear from an interested partner, she contacts him under some small pretext. To be quite frank, she told us, she made herself too available and too easy to seduce. Her new approach now, for she feels she has nothing to lose, is to slow down the courting process. Instead of phoning to speak to her new love interest she is prepared to wait for him to phone her. If he never phones, so be it.

IF HE NEVER PHONES, SO BE IT

Francene's list

Francene is in her late 20s.

1. I have a certain set of lingerie I call my 'lucky undies' which I wear, whether it be on a first date or going somewhere special.

2. I have a certain perfume I prefer to wear, 'Joop Femme'.

3. I always wear my hair out. This makes me feel more relaxed about the way I look.

4. I always wear black. Usually it consists of pants and a top showing some skin between neck and bust. Not too much bust though.

5. I use a lot of eye contact, you know those long, but not too long, stares are great.

6. I always have a smile on my face. I think this is very important, it makes you look like you are fun to be around.

7. I usually try to talk a bit, but not too much.

8. I try to ask lots of questions about them, in the hope that a second date will happen and they can find out more about me then.

9. And finally I have this little laugh I use throughout the date, though I try not to use it too much.

These are my tricks of the trade. Whether they work for anyone else I don't know. I can say they have definitely worked for me because every time I have gone on a date and done these things, I have either scored another one or it has turned into an ongoing relationship.

Peter's list

Peter is in his early 30s.

1. I wear clothes which are modern but stylishly casual on a first date because I prefer to go to a casual restaurant.

2. My grooming is good and I wear aftershave.

3. Either I pick her up from her home, or we meet at the venue. It will not be a pub because that's too noisy, rather, a nice restaurant.

4. I sit opposite her so we can talk easily and so we can see each other's eyes and features well. It makes me more captivating too.

5. I like to ask questions. Then I can sit back and listen.

6. I make good eye contact.

7. My general behaviour is cautious.

8. I only touch if it is appropriate and then very lightly.

9. This is a friendship opportunity. I am not looking for a long-standing thing. I ask myself can I have fun with this person?

10. I don't push the situation sexually.

11. If I take her home I give her a kiss on the cheek. If we part at the restaurant because she has driven there herself, I will also give her a kiss on the cheek.

12. My purpose for the date is to discover her personality and notice her behaviours.

Sarah's list

Sarah is in her early 40s.

1. I behave in a very feminine way, confident yet non-threatening, soft with a quiet strength and assurance.

2. I am happy, a pleasure to be with and good company. I smile and laugh a lot.

3. I always flirt with my eyes. So it means making a lot of eye contact and being very expressive with them.

4. I show a lot of interest in him and his life.

5. I tell him only snippets of information about me, enough to keep him intrigued, while keeping the focus on him. I am not secretive, I just hold back some information for future dates.

6. I wear clothing and colours which flatter me, never brown, grey, beige or all black.

7. I always wear sensual matching underwear which makes me feel sensual, romantic and feminine.

8. I wear subtle make-up and accentuate my eyes.

9. I make sure I am well groomed.

10. I wear a soft floral perfume such as 'Paris' or 'L'Air du Temps'.

11. I always wear jewellery to accentuate my femininity: two or three rings, two bracelets, earrings and a necklace or chain, all in gold or silver, but never garish.

I WEAR CLOTHING AND COLOURS WHICH FLATTER ME

12. On a first date I don't touch much. The most I will do is brush up against him as we walk, sometimes touching his arm as we speak.

13. I don't usually invite him into my home on a first date, either before or after. He comes to my home and we leave straight away.

14. I always wait for him to call me and to make the first moves. I believe men like to be hunters and this gives them a sense of control.

All my first dates have led to more dates or long-term relationships including seven marriage proposals.

Jack's list

Jack is in his late 20s.

1. I love women and have studied how they react to situations with body language over many years.

2. With this in mind I know I have to look good. Women are aware of lots of details about you. I make sure I combine interesting colours well.

3. My grooming is impeccable. I use subtle and expensive aftershave.

4. I usually pick her up from her home or we sometimes meet at a venue.

5. I help her sit down. Women love this.

6. Over dinner in a medium priced restaurant that has style, I ask her about herself. I always get her thinking by asking questions such as: 'what's been your happiest time ever?' or

'what would you change about your life if you could go back in time?'

7. I make sure we smile a lot and laugh often too.
8. I give her my full attention.
9. I praise her appearance and her successes in life.
10. I gently touch her hand as we sit opposite each other.
11. I ask her not to tell me everything about herself – 'Please leave that for next time'.
12. I am always a gentleman, sometimes a very courteous gentleman, sometimes a definite Romeo. It depends on the reaction I have been getting from her all evening. I have to pace my approach.
13. I can wait for sex until another time. If you wait, and work on building the relationship first, the sex has more meaning and passion when it happens.

Women chase me. I am not the best looking man in town, but I do know how to treat women.

DATING TURN-OFFS

It's amazing how many men and women ensure rejection by their choice of behaviours on a first date. Here are some dating turn-offs to avoid :

For women

- stop talking about personal or work problems
- stop criticising ex-boyfriends or husbands
- don't appear too keen
- don't tell him you could fall in love with him

- don't discuss marriage and your dreams about the wedding day
- don't tell your life story
- don't be too secretive
- resist wearing heavy perfume and make-up
- resist freshening up your lipstick and make-up in front of him
- stop yourself asking too many questions about his finances
- don't have so much skin and cleavage exposed that you obviously think your sex appeal is your greatest asset
- don't aim to have sex on the first date

For Men

- don't talk about or criticise previous girlfriends or wives
- stop trying to control the occasion
- stop talking about yourself too much
- resist name dropping and talking about your possessions
- don't dress in an out-of-date way or inappropriately
- don't be poorly groomed
- resist being distracted by every attractive woman passing by
- resist becoming too familiar
- don't drink too much alcohol
- don't expect sex on the first date

What colours should you wear

The choice of clothing and colours relates to what you have in your wardrobe, where you are going, the climate and time of year as well as the image you wish to project. Above all this, you must be comfortable so you can concentrate on your fascinating partner and not have to worry about tight belts, sore feet or being overdressed. Now add to your knowledge by considering the effect of colour on you and a partner.

For the first rendezvous

Choose a colour you know looks good on you. Nothing neutral at this time, rather a colour others compliment you on each time you wear it. It will probably be a colour enhancing your natural colouring. Research shows men are attracted to women wearing peachy/apricot-toned colours or mid-tone blues, so these could be a good choice for women.

CHOOSE A COLOUR YOU KNOW LOOKS GOOD ON YOU

Many women are attracted to turquoise, shades of blue and burgundy. Either of these would be good choices for a man's shirt colour. Interestingly, men tend to undervalue women wearing turquoise, so women should avoid turquoise until their friend has a chance to get to know the real person.

Colours to avoid on the first date

Women should stay away from dressing completely in red since it has overt sexual connotations unless this is their intention. Wearing all pink is too romantic for the first meeting. If you like the sophistication of black, navy, dark brown or dark grey reconsider your thoughts for this occasion. They are daunting and not friendly. A colour which is medium to light is friendly and attractive.

Men should not dress in neutrals. Add some colour. This way you are adding zest. No one wants to be involved with a neutral person. If the first time you go out you are in casual clothes, it is easy to wear a blue, burgundy or some other coloured shirt. If you are wearing a suit, add some colour interest in the tie. Women like patterned ties, so choose a tie with colours in it which complement the jacket and one which is contemporary. Looking up-to-date shows your friend you are a modern man, not one who lives in the past.

AND AS THE RELATIONSHIP DEVELOPS

If choosing neutrals (greys, beiges, black, white or browns) is your preferred style, add the sparkle of colour in your accessories. For men this could be a tie or casual shirt. Add medium colour somewhere near your face especially if you are a play-it-safe person. Break away from the all-blue look, it merely characterises you as conservative and wanting a quiet and calm life.

For women, perhaps add a scarf, earrings or other jewellery or one eye-catching colour in a sweater or casual blouse. Certainly when women wear neutrals, wearing make-up adds the dimension of colour artistry.

For both men and women at this stage there are no preferred colours for getting on well with your new partner, except to say you need medium colours now. Be yourself and let it show. If you prefer black for whatever reason, know you will have to work very hard on the relationship to have closeness. Why not add some colour near your face so you are more approachable.

BE YOURSELF AND LET IT SHOW

The purpose of wearing medium to deep colours at the developing stages of the relationship is to say at conscious and subconscious levels you are excited about being alive. You are not wishy-washy. You are not aloof. You have a colourful life and you are confidently intriguing. If your relationship is moving along happily you are probably feeling more confident within yourself anyway. Express it in your colour choices. There is no better time than now to be a little daring.

For more about what clothes to wear and why, see Chapter 3 'Romancing the Body'.

Where to on the first date?

On a first date, you want to be confident, comfortable and show yourself off to the best advantage. A first date is in many ways like going for a job interview. There, you present yourself in the best light possible, dress in an appropriate manner and hope you say the right words and have the answers to get the job. You feel nervous beforehand and don't know afterwards if the prospective employer finds you acceptable.

So it is the first time you go out with a new love interest. You think carefully about where to go, what to wear and how to behave. You feel nervous beforehand hoping everything goes well. Sometimes you feel like cancelling because the pain or anxiety doesn't seem worth it. Because there is no intimate history between you, the first date is fraught with awkwardness.

Consider the impact of colour psychology within restaurants. Colour isn't everything for the first date but it will certainly have a subconscious effect.

- a restaurant decorated in peach or apricot tones, or with terracotta floor tiles having peach/orange tones as a strong feature, or at least the cloths or serviettes in these colours, encourages conversation and closer communication. These colours are warmer and more romantic than blues and greens.
- A restaurant using a lot of yellow, even though it creates a happy friendly atmosphere could also increase the anxiety of both parties on a first date, or in someone who is tired after a busy day. Come back to it as the romance blossoms. (A yellow decorated venue works very well to stimulate ideas and conversation if a relationship becomes stale later on. It can also add some fun to a romance which may be suffering from being too serious and boring.)

- For the first date stay away from a restaurant which is decorated in red, unless your aim is to have a sexual relationship from the very beginning. Red stimulates the senses enormously. Do you want a long-lasting and romantic relationship? Don't go to bed with your new friend on the first date. Let the relationship develop. Getting to know each other mentally and spiritually before you know each other physically gives you more chance of developing a lasting friendship. Once the flirting reaches a certain level, a red restaurant may be the prelude for your first sexual encounter.
- A restaurant decorated with pinks is not a good idea for the first encounter. It is too romantic. Keep it in mind for later on in the relationship.
- How about blue? No. It's too cool, too contemplative and not stimulating enough for your first rendezvous unless the restaurant uses some warm tones as decorative touches with the blue. If your relationship later has tension in it, blue will help calm and release animosity and anxiety. Turquoise however, has a light-hearted air. It is more suitable at the beginning of the relationship than blue.
- A restaurant decor based on green is relaxing and rejuvenating after a busy day.
- Neutrals perhaps? Look at the cloths and napkins used to enliven the white, beige, cream or grey walls. Notice the colour of the plates, the flooring and the wall decorations. What you are aiming for is something warm and inviting and most important, conducive to conversation. Is the food and its presentation important? Of course but as is the way with intimacy, food becomes almost secondary to the emotional communication.

Keep the first occasion you spend time together light-hearted and comfortable for both of you. Here are some safe choices for the first rendezvous:

- A coffee shop to have a cup of something and a good chat.
- A restaurant, but consider the mood the restaurant of your choice creates. Choose carefully not only for the food, setting or the convenient location but also for the colour scheme. Yes, we are serious! Lighting is important too. Don't choose a restaurant with strong or harsh lighting. And don't forget music. Too loud and you won't be able to speak.
- The movies. To avoid embarrassment, choose a middle-of-the-road film which is not too violent, nor too romantic. Comedies are probably the right choice. Keep everything light-hearted for a first date. No demands, no heavy philosophical discussion and no detailed revelations about your life. Don't suggest watching a video at their place or yours. You both need others around you for comfort and security on a first date.
- Fun parks can bring out the child in you both.
- Sailing can be a very relaxing and enjoyable first date.
- The beach is great for a walk or a swim.
- A drive in the country.
- An art gallery or tourist attraction is a good choice but check first that your passion for these entertainments is enjoyed by your partner too.
- A sports event.
- A dinner or party with friends.

KEEP THE FIRST OCCASION YOU SPEND TIME TOGETHER LIGHT HEARTED

There is a common thread with all these rendezvous. There are other people around. It is important you develop this component. Then you will observe how your friend behaves in public, you will both have interesting distractions involving others' activities and you will both feel safely confident.

Romance takes careful consideration.

CHAPTER 3
romancing the body
... colour, sex, clothes and you

They had agreed to meet at a coffee shop after he answered her personal advertisement in a newspaper. On the telephone they seemed to have a lot in common. She thought he sounded intelligent, friendly and approachable. She knew what to wear for this first important meeting. She knew that dressy casual would give the message she desired. Not over the top, she thought, yet showing a style which summed up her attitude to life. After all she had described herself as a 'stylish redhead with a definite flair for looking good, seeking the company of a well-educated non-smoking optimist, late 40s to 50s. Must enjoy a comfortable and sophisticated lifestyle, have a good sense of humour and a heavy dose of enthusiasm.'

Imagine Carolyn's surprise when Tony met her wearing faded jeans, plaid shirt and scuffed boots. Immediately she rejected him as a potential partner. If this was the best he could do when first impressions count, there was no way Carolyn wanted to develop the relationship. She knew appearance wasn't everything and he seemed reasonably pleasant, but why hadn't he read her advertisement with more insight? If she had emphasised appearance as the first thing on the list describing herself, why had he turned up for the first encounter looking scruffy?

Some people just don't understand the power of the first impression. Many men and women haven't worked out how to look most attractive for themselves and for a partner. Perhaps it's a confidence issue. Perhaps it reflects a view that appearance isn't everything. We've news for you. Non-verbal behaviour influences others much more than words do. Be sure you think through carefully your clothing and grooming choices. They are powerful aspects of non-verbal behaviour. Make a positive first impression.

SOME PEOPLE JUST DON'T UNDERSTAND THE POWER OF THE FIRST IMPRESSION

Here are some tips to help you when you are searching for the perfect partner. When you follow these ideas you will gain confidence and insight. First we'll look at outer wear for men and women. Then we'll hold your hand as we introduce you to the Colour and Sensuality Quotient factor of underwear. Initially we look at new romance situations, then we move on to information for those of you who have already found the love of your life.

Outer wear

Use the concept of 'less is more' when considering accessories, flamboyance and pattern. If there is too much texture, pattern and jewellery to distract your new friend, how can he or she concentrate on you? Take a look in a full-length mirror to check the balance of accessories and colour.

And what about your new friend? Your first date is your opportunity to gain a sense of your friend's grooming and whether they satisfy your sense of visual attractiveness and basic appearance criteria. Here at first hand is your opportunity to check the details.

MEN AND WOMEN ON A FIRST DATE

The question is: what do you want to achieve?
* Sex on the first date?
* You don't want sex at the end of this first outing?
* You do want to arouse interest for possible romance and sex in the future?
* You can't read the future but want to present as attractively as possible?
* Your self-esteem wants you to always look attractive and appropriately dressed?
* Or there is some other agenda?

Men

What you wear on this first date depends on where you are going. Think it through. Visualise what most people at the venue would be wearing. A good tip is to dress the same level as the other people around you or one level above. Women are tremendously impressed by men who understand colour coordination. If you have difficulty with this, ask a friend for help. Women very rarely tell you when you have made a mess with colours, they store the knowledge away and hope to see an improvement next time, or come to the conclusion you may well be poorly coordinated in other areas of your personal life too.

WOMEN ARE TREMENDOUSLY IMPRESSED BY MEN WHO UNDERSTAND COLOUR COORDINATION

Ensure the colours blend and don't compete. When in doubt, choose the safest path and have variations of a colour theme, for example blues, from pale through to dark. Grey trousers or jacket go well with black with a vibrant colour added for interest. This is another option which may suit you. For ideas on colour combinations look in a few menswear shop windows or fashion magazines.

The more structured your choice of clothing, the more business-like you will appear. Depending on the circumstances, it may be appropriate to soften your business look by wearing a coloured shirt. The world loves men in blue shirts with a suit. Add a bright tie or one with a bigger and bolder pattern than normal. Your tie choice expresses your personality more than any other business clothing choice. Enjoy either a repeated geometric pattern, which will give the appearance of structure, or curves in the pattern which suggests you are creative. Medium colours work well too.

Only wear a T-shirt if you are meeting very casually. A collared knit shirt or polo shirt works much better. The collar lifts you from very casual to smarter casual.

Wear a sweater only if the circumstances seem appropriate. The rule of thumb is, if the surroundings are casual, a sweater is fine. If the surroundings are more formal or you want to impress, a jacket is better. If you want to hide your heavy stomach, never wear a sweater. It clings too closely.

Grooming makes all the difference to the first impression. Here are some tips for success:
- Go lightly with aftershave, very lightly. You don't even have to wear it.
- Use a deodorant.
- Be very clean. No spots or stains on your tie or trousers, no blood on your collar from shaving, no grubby cuffs.
- Don't wear a shirt which shows sweat stains under the arms.
- Have clean well-cut nails.

- Have your hair under control, but don't use too much gel or mousse. Your hair should look touchable.
- If you don't go regularly to the hairdresser shave the back of the neck so it is clean .
- Shave the front of your neck low enough to stop hair tufts peeking over the shirt collar.
- Have clean shoes, well polished if leather.
- Tie your tie to the correct length (just over the belt buckle).
- Keep your shirt tucked in.
- Don't adjust your genitals in public. This is gross behaviour.

Are women fussy? Yes. Do they notice details? You'd better believe it.

The fit of a man's clothes is very important to a woman. She notices every detail.

Women admire:
* The correct length of trousers, not too long and in particular, not too short.
* You, when you wear your belt on your waist line, not on your hips.
* You, when you wear a belt. Don't think you can get away with not having one.
* The collar of your shirt fitting properly. It is not a good look to be pulling at your collar constantly. It is not a good look for you to have the top button of your shirt undone behind your tie.
* You, when your shirt fits your torso well. No straining, and no popped buttons please.
* The fact you know how to buy a jacket to fit your shoulders well.

* The fact you know how to buy trousers to fit your backside well.

WOMEN ARE IMPRESSED WITH SMOOTH-FITTING CLOTHES

Women are impressed with smooth-fitting clothes. Smooth does not mean tight. Even though you have pockets, don't put much in them. This includes coins and keys, handkerchiefs and bulky wallets. Why change the shape of one of your most interesting physical assets? Women always check out the shape of men's backsides to see how well the trousers fit. Smooth is sensual.

Women

Less is more in terms of jewellery, perfume and make-up. The circumstances, climate, venue and time of day will determine what you wear. Remember our tip about dressing the same level or only one level above. It really works. Avoid a business look unless you are going straight from work to the rendezvous. Even so, you need to lighten and loosen the business look a little.

Colour works for or against you. Black, grey, dark brown are all aloof colours. They give you control but don't tell him much about you. Many women use black as a constant cover-up. It is sophisticated and alluring when you have some skin showing, but not, for day wear, very welcoming.

The styles you choose should be flattering and a little sensual. Show some skin, just not too much. What you wear, more than what he wears, sets the scene. If you prefer slacks, wear them. If you prefer a short skirt, wear it. Realise the more skin you show, on arms, legs, body, thighs and even feet, the more sexually

LEAVE SOME MYSTERY FOR THE NEXT ENCOUNTER

inviting you appear. You don't have to go to the other extreme, just leave some mystery for the next encounter. Let your femininity shine through.

Here are some grooming tips to help you:
- Be careful with your perfume. Most men like some, but don't put on too much. It is better to apply it on your body lightly before getting dressed rather than on wrists and neck.
- If you use hair spray, choose a brand with very little or no scent. It adds too much if you are already wearing perfume. Your hair must look relaxed and even touchable. Hair that moves is alluring to men.
- Wear a deodorant.
- Brush the stray hairs off your shoulders before meeting your friend. If your hair is long, don't fiddle with it as you speak.
- Men admire women who wear subtle make-up. Enhance your eyes, your lips and your skin and never apply foundation thickly. Attempting to cover up freckles and lines doesn't work.
- Have immaculate nails which are not too long. Men like refined, natural and well-shaped nails, so bright reds and oranges are out.
- Choose clothes which fit you properly. No bursting buttons or skirts you know are too tight or too big.
- Check your bra strap isn't showing and that you don't have to adjust your straps in front of him.
- Men don't like jewellery junkies. If your preferred style is to wear a lot of jewellery we don't want to change you. Just limit the number for the first date. It is more important that you are the focus – not the jewellery. Invest in quality. If you wear large earrings cut back on the other jewellery.

- Check the appearance of your stockings, and their coordination with your shoes and hemline.

LATER IN A RELATIONSHIP

Your relationship may be months or years old. Don't give up on appearance and good grooming. Keep looking your best and take the trouble to present yourself well at all times, not only when you go out as a couple. There is nothing surer to sour the romance than you not taking pride in your appearance. You would also be telegraphing to your lover and the world, that you are taking the relationship for granted. Slop around at weekends when that's appropriate. Everyone loves to relax wearing really comfortable clothes. Keep an eye on how your partner presents at these times. Tatty or neat? Make a compromise gesture so you both feel at ease.

When you have a special time planned for your partner, dress up. Imagine you are in the romancing and courting phase again. When you are on show as a couple don't always wear conservative or very neutral coloured clothing. Be adventurous occasionally. Look to put some zing in your life. Develop the adventurous spirit by thinking about gifts of accessories and contemporary clothing for yourself and your lover. Keep up to date with what's happening in fashion and hair styling. This process will allow you to see the world and your relationship through contemporary eyes. The saddest path is for both of you to become more and more conservative in your appearance and behaviour. Polishing up your appearance is uplifting to your spirit and your sensuality.

> **POLISHING UP YOUR APPEARANCE IS UPLIFTING TO YOUR SPIRIT AND YOUR SENSUALITY**

Underwear

Your choice of underwear is one of the strongest indicators of your sensuality and your emotionally romantic state. We have interviewed owners and assistants in lingerie boutiques, men's and women's underwear suppliers, and interested male and female participants to arrive at an appraisal of what we call the intimate **Colour and Sensuality Quotient (CSQ)**. This completely new concept will have you thinking carefully about what you wear each day, and when you want to be sensual and seductive. To determine the male CSQ we spent long hours examining and discussing men's underpants in shops and with manufacturers. We compared 20 pairs of underpants, all of different colours and styles to consider the sensuality quotients. To test our theories, we spoke to many women about our findings. Everyone's imagination ran riot.

> **YOUR CHOICE OF UNDERWEAR IS ONE OF THE STRONGEST INDICATORS OF YOUR SENSUALITY**

Looking at women's underwear took even longer because there are so many choices and combinations possible. Again we examined dozens of examples of women's underwear. We sought opinions from men, and then we got the facts from buyers who told us what women buy for themselves, and what men buy for women.

The CSQ appraisal is based on the reaction of men to women's underwear – colours, fabrics and styles; and women's reaction to men's underwear – colours, fabrics and styles. The CSQ can be sobering. You might think you are putting on sensual, attractive underwear, and discover, when you do the CSQ quiz, that you score only 4 out of 10.

The Colour and Sensuality Quotient

There are some important points to be considered as you do your own CSQ quiz:

- A score of 7 or more out of 10 means you are wearing sensual underwear.
- You don't have to wear some of the top scoring styles if they don't suit your body shape. You can still be very sensual without achieving the perfect 10.
- Underwear and clothes aren't everything. You could have a score of 9 for your CSQ and yet not be sensually seductive because of your body language or conversation. Be sure the three mix well.
- Women who prefer cotton can stay with it for most days, and introduce one sexy underwear combination with some polyester or lycra with a cotton gusset, for special occasions.
- Tomato or true red is the colour of sex: blatant sex. If provocative sex is what you desire, choose it. This colour is associated with eroticism, striptease, prostitution and one-night stands. It you desire the passion and lust associated with red, plus some control, choose a slightly deeper red such as burgundy or a red wine colour.

> **TOMATO OR TRUE RED IS THE COLOUR OF SEX: BLATANT SEX**

- Styles, fashion and fabrics change so quickly. Whatever appears in the future will still fit the stereotype of sensual underwear. CSQ hasn't changed in centuries. It is, after all about skin, concealment, colour and texture.
- For men's CSQ we have only included underpants. Women don't regard singlets as sexy. You may look good in a skimpy top teamed with underpants but for CSQ reasons we can't count it.

- CSQ is important for men's underwear. However in our society it's women's underwear which is regarded as being more sensual. The undressing of a woman's body is usually a more provocative process for a man than for a woman.
- Very few men or women dress sensually every day. On practical days, your score could be a 3. Our CSQ is for those special times when you know you want to be confident in your sexiness and sensuality. We can promise you though, once you begin working out your CSQ on a daily basis, it will strongly influence your underwear purchases forever.
- Have fun shopping for sensual underwear.

HAVE FUN SHOPPING FOR SENSUAL UNDERWEAR

MEN'S UNDERPANTS

Remember that your CSQ is based on colour and sensuality through a woman's eyes not a man's. To calculate your CSQ, give yourself a score out of 10 for each of the three factors: **colour**, **fabric** and **style**. Arrive at your score out of a possible 30, having scored out of 10 for each of the three categories. Then divide by 3. This will be your CSQ score out of 10.

For example:
* A man who wears red cotton knit hipsters will score: 10+5+9 = 24. Then divide 24 by 3 to reach a CSQ of 8.
* A man who wears deep blue polyester satin boxers, scores 3+9+5 = 17 which divided by 3 gives him a CSQ of 5.6.
* A man who wears black cotton knit fitted boxers, scores 8+5+8 = 21 which divided by 3 gives him a CSQ of 7.
* A man who wears navy cotton knit Y-front briefs, scores 3+5+2 = 10 which divided by 3 gives him a CSQ of 3.3.

A CSQ score of 7 or more means you are wearing sensual underpants.

Colour	Rating out of 10
True/Tomato Red	10
Burgundy Red	10
Black	8
Various Purples	7
Turquoise	6
Light Blue	5
White	4
Dark Green, Deep Blue and Navy	3
Brights, and Orange, Gold, Hot Pink, Lime	3
Beige	2
Mustard	1
Grey	1

Remember that brights represent surprise elements and are fun. Patterned underpants should be rated according to the predominant colour. If there are two major colours, for example red and white, score 10 for red and 4 for white and average that out to 7 as your colour rating. Patterns are not as sensual as plain unless they have erotic elements in the pattern.

Fabric	Rating out of 10
Shiny Lycra	10
Polyester Satin	9
Silk	9
Matte Lycra (Stretchy)	8
Cotton and Lycra (Slightly Stretchy)	6
Cotton Knit	5
Woven Cotton (Like Shirt Material)	3

STYLE	RATING OUT OF 10
G-STRING	10
NARROW SIDED HIPSTER (STRING BIKINI)	10
HIPSTER	9
COTTON KNIT, FITTED BOXER	8
BOXER	5
SUPPORT BRIEF	2
Y-FRONT BRIEF	2
'TENT' BOXER	1

How did you score?

WOMEN'S UNDERWEAR

We have identified six components for women's underwear CSQ. This means that, unlike a man who divides his final total out of 30 by 3 to come to his CSQ, a woman has a total out of 60 and needs to divide her score by 6 to reach her CSQ out of 10. We look at the colour, fabric and style of bras then the colour, fabric and style of pants.

- Pants include panties, knickers or briefs. These last two are used as follows: French knickers – those loose-legged smooth fabric pants which have become popular once more; briefs – the plain pants which fit a woman to the waist.
- Bikinis are narrow-sided pants. They can be high cut or ordinary cut.
- Push up bras are bras padded underneath (usually with extra inserts) to push the breasts up and, by creating uplift, make the breasts seem larger.
- A padded bra is lightly padded all over to give fullness.
- Body suits and teddies are all in one underwear garments worn instead of bra and pants. The body suit which is a structured

one-piece garment with a bra, is worn under clothing or under jackets as a top in its own right. Men score them super high. There are two types: one with G-string, and the other with normal backside covering. Often the latter will have detachable suspenders. The teddy is an all-in-one soft garment with no structured bra, usually decorated with lace and looking like sleep wear.

- A general guide for all women's underwear is: shiny is more sensual than matte; lacy is more sensual than plain; sheer is more sensual than solid.
- Black is the most popular for women's underwear in the eyes of men in the Western world because of its mystery, sophistication and seduction factors. At another level it is popular with women too because black always means 'control'. Women need to feel control over their sexuality. In a long-term relationship, black can become boring because the surprise element has disappeared. Occasionally wear red or even white.

WOMEN NEED TO FEEL CONTROL OVER THEIR SEXUALITY

- The two reds mentioned are not as popular as black or white with women because of the overt sexuality. There is no denying that the reds are sensually stimulating colours. That's why they score 10.
- White may surprise you when you compare it with the score for men's white. White underwear on a woman suggests purity, a fresh start, even new beginnings. A man seeing white on a woman often desires that, no matter how new or old the relationship. This is a subconscious reaction.
- Skin- or flesh-coloured underwear may well be a favourite for women because it is practical and can be worn under light coloured clothing. Some women also think it is sexy because

a woman wearing just flesh-coloured or beige underwear looks nude but men don't agree. They like to have their imagination teased by seeing a distinct difference between skin and underwear colour.
* Bright colours score reasonably well because they are a surprise and bring an element of fun into sensuality.

Remember your CSQ is based on colour and sensuality through a man's eyes not a woman's.

To calculate your CSQ give yourself a score out of 10 for each of the three factors: **colour**, **fabric** and **style** for bras and then a score out of 10 for each of the three factors: **colour**, **fabric** and **style** for pants. There is separate advice on how to score the CSQ of body suits and teddies.

Arrive at your score out of a possible 60, having scored out of 10 for each of the 6 categories. Then divide by 6 to reach your CSQ score out of 10.

For example:
* A woman who wears a black, see-through lacy with no sheen, low cut bra scores 10+9+9 = 28. If she adds to it a black, see-through lacy with sheen, high cut bikini pant, she scores 10+10+ 9 = 29. Total out of 60 = 57. Then divide 57 by 6 to reach a CSQ of 9.5.
* A woman who wears a beige, see-through lacy with some sheen, half-cup bra scores 3+10+10 = 23. If she adds pants which are beige, see-through lacy with no sheen bikini she scores 3+9+7 = 19. Total out of 60 =42. Then divide 42 by 6 to reach a CSQ of 7.
* A woman who wears a white, matte and lacy, half-cup push up bra scores 8+6+10 = 24. If she adds a white, matte and

lacy, G-string she scores 8+6+10 = 24. Total out of 60 = 48. Divide 48 by 6 to reach a CSQ of 8.

* A woman who wears a white, satin finish, full-cup bra scores 8+4+5 = 17. If she adds pink, see-through lacy with no sheen, briefs she scores 6+9+3 = 18. Total out of 60 = 35. Deduct 2 points for bra and pants not matching in colour and 1 point for them not matching in fabric at all. (See information on these deductions after Body Suits and Teddies). The score then becomes 32. Divide 32 by 6 to reach a CSQ of 5.3.

A CSQ score of 7 or more means you are wearing sensual underwear.

BRAS

COLOUR	RATING OUT OF 10
TRUE RED	10
BURGUNDY	10
BLACK	10
WHITE (SOFT WHITE TO IVORY, NOT CREAM)	8
PURPLES (MULBERRY, GRAPE, AUBERGINE, PLUM)	7
PINK	6
ORANGE AND GOLD	5
BLUE (LIGHT TO DEEP) AND DENIM LOOK	5
PEACH, APRICOT, CREAM	4
GREENS, BEIGE, MOCHA, CHAMPAGNE, BROWN	3
GREY	2
FABRIC	**RATING OUT OF 10**
SEE-THROUGH LACY WITH SOME SHEEN	10
SEE-THROUGH LACY WITH NO SHEEN	9
SEE-THROUGH	8
LACY WITH SOME SHEEN (NOT SEE THROUGH)	7

	Rating out of 10
SATIN/SILK WITH LACE	7
MATTE AND LACY	6
MATTE WITH SHEEN PATTERN	6
LACY COTTON (eg BRODERIE ANGLAIS)	5
SATIN FINISH	4
STRETCH COTTON	3
COTTON	2
MATTE	2

Style	**Rating out of 10**
HALF-CUP INCLUDING PUSH UP	10
LOW-CUT INCLUDING PUSH UP	9
PADDED HALF-CUP	8
FULL-CUP	5
PADDED FULL-CUP	5
SPORTS	2
CAMISOLE (INSTEAD OF BRA)	4

Pants

Colour	**Rating out of 10**
TRUE RED	10
BURGUNDY	10
BLACK	10
WHITE (SOFT WHITE TO IVORY, NOT CREAM)	8
PURPLES (MULBERRY, GRAPE, AUBERGINE, PLUM)	7
PINK	6
ORANGE AND GOLD	5
BLUE (LIGHT TO DEEP) AND DENIM LOOK	5
PEACH, APRICOT, CREAM	4
GREENS, BEIGE, MOCHA, CHAMPAGNE, BROWN	3
GREY	2

Fabric	Rating out of 10
SEE-THROUGH LACY WITH SOME SHEEN	10
SEE-THROUGH LACY WITH NO SHEEN	9
SEE-THROUGH	8
LACY WITH SOME SHEEN (NOT SEE THROUGH)	7
SATIN/SILK WITH LACE	7
MATTE AND LACY	6
MATTE WITH SHEEN PATTERN	6
LACY COTTON (eg BRODERIE ANGLAIS)	5
SATIN FINISH	4
STRETCH COTTON	3
COTTON	2
MATTE	2

Style	Rating out of 10
G-STRING AND STRING BIKINI	10
HIGH CUT BIKINI	9
FRENCH KNICKERS (LOOSE-LEGGED)	8
BIKINI	7
HIGH CUT BRIEFS	7
BRIEFS	3
WOMEN'S BOXERS	2

Body suits and teddies

Colour	Rating out of 10
TRUE RED	10
BURGUNDY	10
BLACK	10
WHITE (SOFT WHITE TO IVORY, NOT CREAM)	8
PURPLES (MULBERRY, GRAPE, AUBERGINE, PLUM)	7
PINK	6

ORANGE AND GOLD	5
BLUE (LIGHT TO DEEP) AND DENIM LOOK	5
PEACH, APRICOT, CREAM	4
GREENS, BEIGE, MOCHA, CHAMPAGNE, BROWN	3
GREY	2

FABRIC	**RATING OUT OF 10**
SEE-THROUGH LACY WITH SOME SHEEN	10
SEE-THROUGH LACY WITH NO SHEEN	9
SEE-THROUGH	8
LACY WITH SOME SHEEN (NOT SEE THROUGH)	7
SATIN/SILK WITH LACE	7
MATTE AND LACY	6
MATTE WITH SHEEN PATTERN	6
LACY COTTON (eg BRODERIE ANGLAIS)	5
SATIN FINISH	4
STRETCH COTTON	3
COTTON	2
MATTE	2

STYLE	**RATING OUT OF 10**
BODY SUIT WITH FITTED BRA AND G-STRING	10
BODY SUIT WITH FITTED BRA	9
BODY SUIT WITH FITTED BRA AND SUSPENDERS	9
BODY SUIT WITH NO FITTED BRA, BUT G-STRING	9
TEDDY WITH NO UNDERWEAR STRUCTURE	8

Once you have your score out of 30 for body suits and teddies, you will need to double it to have a score out of 60. Then divide that score by 6. These body suits and teddies take the place of bras and pants.

Important extra information:

- If you wear suspenders and stockings in the same colour as your underwear, **add 3 points** to your score out of 60. Then divide by 6 for the final CSQ score.
- If you wear suspenders and stockings in a different colour from your underwear, **add 2 points** to your score out of 60. Then divide by 6 for the final CSQ score.
- If you don't wear a bra give yourself **a score of 20 out of 30 for bra colour, fabric and style**. Skin is sensual, but mystery is more intriguing for men.
- If you don't wear a bra but do wear a camisole instead, you will find your colour, fabric and style score easily under the bra list.
- If your pants and bra don't match in colour, **deduct 2 points** from your score out of 60 before dividing by 6.
- If your pants and bra are totally different in pattern or fabric from each other, **deduct 1 point** from your score out of 60 before dividing by 6. (Use your common sense with this. A bra which is see-through lacy with some sheen, for example, teamed with high cut briefs which are see-through lacy with no sheen won't lose a point. They are not totally different.)

Nightwear

Many of the same principles apply to nightwear. For women, look at how much skin is exposed, and consider the colour of the fabric and the style of the nightgown or pyjamas, or whatever you wear. Remember that mystery is much more intriguing than nakedness, particularly in the early stages of seduction.

REMEMBER THAT MYSTERY IS MUCH MORE INTRIGUING THAN NAKEDNESS

For men, mystery is the key too. A man wearing something over his genitals is more intriguing than him parading around the house naked. Once you are in bed that's a very different story. Nudity is all the go then.

> Your choice of underwear is one of the strongest indicators of your sensuality and your emotionally romantic state.

CHAPTER 4

the biology of sex

... colourful body, colourful seduction

Our outlook on life changes when lust and love become the central focus. The body physiology also alters when we experience feelings of desire and lust. Well-known zoologist, Desmond Morris described human beings as the sexiest primates alive. In *The Human Animal*, he stated that 'despite the different skin colours, beliefs and rituals to be found in the 5000 million human beings alive today, we actually share an almost identical genetic heritage ... and different courtship rituals across the world reflect the universal emotion of love'.

For humans, the courting processes are different from those performed by other animals. Our closest biological relatives, animals in the monkey family, take a little time to decide on a loved one also. 'People are always surprised when we tell them that orang-utans don't just mate whenever and with whoever they like,' a zookeeper at Sydney's Taronga Zoo said recently. 'It's not wham, bam, thank you ma'am. They have to like each other and get on well, otherwise it just won't happen.'

ARRIVING AT SEXUAL CLOSENESS IS COMPLEX

Arriving at sexual closeness for humans is even more complex and certainly influenced by social customs in each culture. Sexual attraction is based on the power of the five senses. Let's examine each in turn.

Visual appearance

This is our first interest. We glance and then look more closely at the details of the person in our sights. Since all of us have a 'wish list' of preferred appearance locked away in the subconscious, this is the time we check through the possibilities. At heart we are flexible, but we all have some appearance criteria which must be met – fat, thin, plump, well-muscled, short, tall, a certain age, a certain intelligence level, reserved or outgoing and so on. Some of you may say that you don't choose someone by such criteria, as personality is more important. Yes it is. Yet deep down you know what you like the look of. You have had the experience of a physical and chemical attraction to someone before and stored the information away, ready to be retrieved at any time.

If you develop desire for someone who has one major visual annoyance for you, you will accept it initially since there are more important things on hand. You know that you shouldn't judge someone on looks alone. But when the glory and the passion of desire has waned, the physical annoyance may haunt you and may well cause unhappiness.

A word of common sense. When you fall in love, make sure from the beginning that the look and presence of your beloved *takes your breath away*. Perhaps not someone else's breath, because we are not all looking for movie stars as partners, but *your* breath.

WHEN YOU FALL IN LOVE, MAKE SURE FROM THE BEGINNING THAT THE LOOK AND PRESENCE OF YOUR BELOVED *TAKES YOUR BREATH AWAY*

Then those looks and those feelings will warm you on cold nights and comfort you when your beloved is away.

Why are we attracted first by appearance? Because that's where all primates receive their sexual clues. Primal urges flow strongly. What do our closest primate cousins, monkeys, do when wanting a partner? They examine closely and sniff out a rear end of utmost fascination. At backside level any male monkey can tell if the object of his desire is female and is ready to mate.

PRIMAL URGES FLOW STRONGLY

Fortunately, men and women don't show off backsides in that way. We walk upright, but according to zoologists, we have compensated for not having an exposed rear end by developing a new kind of appearance. The rump muscles became better developed so we could walk tall. This meant the backsides of both men and women became muscled, rounded buttocks, something no other primates have.

WOMEN ... SEEING IS BELIEVING

Desmond Morris has suggested a change occurred in female anatomy to compensate for the lack of exposed rear end view. He and others believe the female body developed imitation buttocks at the front, in the form of breasts, which were not only feeding mechanisms but also a powerful sexual signal for males. Morris maintains the female breasts evolved quite simply as buttock mimics. 'So the basic female sexual signal of our species consists of paired fleshy hemispheres.' Rounded at the back and the front!

The undeniable curves of a woman are a highly visual attraction for men. Four areas in particular repeat the curve: the backside, breasts, shoulders and knees. Yes it is true. The shoulders and knees of women are curvy and sexy! Just think how clothing and women's behaviour work towards exposing each one of these.

Recent research also indicates that women reveal more curves and bare flesh when they are ovulating. The reproductive urge obviously doesn't know about contraception.

THE UNDENIABLE CURVES OF A WOMAN ARE A HIGHLY VISUAL ATTRACTION FOR MEN

The backside

Women want jeans, slacks and shorts to fit well especially if they have an attractive backside. Don't underestimate the appeal of the full and curved rear end. Many men are fascinated by the way those two hemispheres move. Because there is more fat and less muscle on women's backsides compared with men's, the movement can be very pronounced. Most women don't want rock and roll effects at their backside. They all seem to know however, that making the hips sway as they walk will attract a man's attention. The swinging, swaying walk is practised by women all over the world and emphasised by mannequins on the catwalk. Women continue the flirtation as they prepare to sit on a chair. The most sensual women move their backsides and hips to position themselves above the chair or lounge then sensually seat themselves.

The breasts

From movies to magazine photos, from cosmetic surgery to breast exercises, from underwear to see-through tops, from wet T-shirt parades to padded bras, women's breasts are the most worked on, worked over, uplifted and exposed body organ in our society. Women's breasts are the wonderful visual difference for men, and women know it and exploit it. Modest women never show cleavage. The less modest will show cleavage and/or nipples through tight or revealing clothing. Remember, however, that the look of the breasts changes with fashion. In the 1950s, breasts were strongly uplifted and pushed out. Today, although the push up bra does big business, the look of breasts under clothing is more natural. Fabrics have helped the change, as have fashion ideas which reveal bare breasts through filmy material. Women know men love their breasts. One of the results of this is an increase in sales in breast firming creams and the number of breast enhancement operations.

WOMEN KNOW MEN LOVE THEIR BREASTS

The shoulders

When women expose their shoulders, in strapless tops, swimming costumes, evening dresses, negligees etc, it is sensual. They are inviting the touch of a hand on their very exposed skin, beginning at the shoulder. The smoothness of the skin on shoulders cannot be overestimated. This is an area where men can begin the sensual touching which may ultimately lead to seduction. Many men find it seductive when an exposed shoulder strap slips off a shoulder. Sensual women know they shouldn't be in too much of a hurry to straighten the strap. The sexiest thing is to let it be. The slipped strap could be the first step to undressing.

The knees

Women's knees are curvier than men's. They may not be your number one turn-on, but fashion regularly exposes these curves with short skirts, shorts and skirt slits. Think how often women cross their legs when seated and show a smooth curved knee. Women also know the crossed leg with exposed thigh is powerful. This is one reason mini skirts have always been successful. There are many 'leg men' who find well-shaped and good-looking women's legs the most attractive part of her anatomy. The curves of a woman's leg, including the shape of the knee, repeat the total curve of the female body. The muscles of the calf, the curve of the instep on the foot, the curve of the upper thigh and the smoothness of these areas emphasised by smooth soft skin and hosiery which flatters, are all seductive.

Men seem to have a preference for a particular part of a woman's anatomy when sexual excitement is on the agenda. They can be divided into three categories:
* leg men
* bum men
* breast men

These are the body areas that turn them on and with which they make superficial judgments of women. Others are influenced by two out of these three, and some men like all areas of a woman's body. A woman knows the area of her body which fascinates the man in her life or a potential lover, simply by observing and remembering where his hands move to when seduction begins. Of course, many men will tell you it is the overall impression that counts, including personality, her way of expression and her outlook on life. Nevertheless breasts, legs and backsides are areas of the female body which are noticed in public and many women, with their choice of clothing, emphasise them deliberately.

Genitals and lips

Unlike other animals, where the display of a female's genitals is the attraction for the mate, human genitals are concealed. Again, Morris suggests, they needed an echo, some form of body mimicry, to transmit a genital signal that could be seen by an approaching man. The answer he suggests are the human lips. Colour them red. Colour them pink. Colour them tones of brown. Apply natural gloss. Make them shiny. All these devices unconsciously mimic and emphasise in a socially acceptable way the female genitals. The increasing popularity of collagen and silicon lip implants are the result of this knowledge. They give the appearance of fuller lips. Perhaps they also subconsciously suggest a sexier woman since, during sexual arousal, lips become engorged with blood making them larger and redder, as does the hidden labia. Choosing lipstick in unnatural colours such as black, purple or bright orange, does not create a sexy look – genitals don't look like that. The glistening, moist and creamy look on lips is chosen for cheesecake photos, because that look mimics aroused genitals. What message does the newer matte lipstick give? Not sexy, but certainly in control of her sexuality.

DURING SEXUAL AROUSAL, LIPS BECOME ENGORGED WITH BLOOD MAKING THEM LARGER AND REDDER

MEN ... SEEING IS BELIEVING

The backsides of men also became rounder, more muscled and tighter, so they could walk upright when the change from being a four-legged to a two-legged animal was complete. There was no need to produce enlarged breasts for men. There is a body shape silhouette difference between the sexes which is very apparent. A man's body has broader shoulders and chest and more strength in the arms than a woman's. Women are instinctively interested in the curves, smoothness and strength which come with muscle formation in men. The curves of men and women are very different and to some extent related to the differences in the body tissue between the sexes. The average male body has 15 per cent fat. The average female body, 28 per cent.

Women are also attracted to the other physiological changes they interpret as representing masculinity: the deeper voice, the hairy face, the hairier body, the squarer jaw, as well as larger hands and feet.

What visual appearance factors do women notice about men? Women do a quick appraisal of their understanding of colour coordination and harmony, grooming, and fit of clothing, including how well the trousers fit his rear end. Individually and in groups women watch men walk by. They notice backsides and whether trousers are too tight, too loose, too low in the crotch or just right. Women notice visual details men wouldn't believe. And they are slow to tell you of their findings. They store the information away to compare it with their appearance wish list. They will decide in your favour if you match 75 per cent of their visual expectation list.

WOMEN NOTICE VISUAL DETAILS MEN WOULDN'T BELIEVE

The sound of the voice and the choice of language

You've checked out your new love interest visually; now you are ready to move to the second criterion for partner picking. Once the mouth opens and the words tumble out, the opportunity is ripe to positively support your choice, or rule out that person. Voice is one of the most important factors affecting the perception you have of others. 'It's not

VOICE IS ONE OF THE MOST IMPORTANT FACTORS AFFECTING THE PERCEPTION YOU HAVE OF OTHERS

what you say but how you say it' movie star and vamp, Mae West stated long ago. Behavioural researchers Loretta Malandro and Larry Barker in their book *Nonverbal Communication* say 'the minute you begin to speak, your spoken image becomes dominant and overrides your visual image. When you talk to someone you can either destroy or reinforce the non-verbal messages you are sending via your clothing, gestures, facial expression, posture and other nonverbal communication.'

Be yourself as you speak. Remember that it may not be the way you say your words or your voice that is unattractive but actually what you are saying. Potential turn-offs are:
* being self-centred and using too many 'I' statements
* talking so much you don't have time to listen
* topics not interesting to your partner: don't be an insensitive bore
* not understanding the art of asking questions

Scent signalling

The third consideration for choosing your beloved is scent. You may have noticed the aftershave or the perfume already, but the *real* smell of the partner's body is only available to you with continuing intimacy. It can be the wonderful mix of savoury and/or sweet which, when your heightened senses notice it during the later stages of courtship, is in itself a turn-on. The smell of another's skin, hair and body lays scent signals to arouse the other senses. They are comforting. They evoke memories even years later. Being up close and personal with the partner you adore means you absorb the smell

THE *REAL* SMELL OF THE PARTNER'S BODY IS ONLY AVAILABLE TO YOU WITH CONTINUING INTIMACY

of their facial skin very readily and reinforces the pleasurable feelings and emotions each time you access the intimacy.

Ensure your body and hair smell clean and fresh. Hair tufts trap the natural fragrance of the body, under arms, around the chest of men and in the genital areas. On clean bodies the natural scents are very erotic but layers of clothing make the natural smell deteriorate and become stale. Most people choose antiperspirants under arms with the understanding that no smell is better than a good smell gone bad.

The perfume/fragrance industry has grown rapidly. Women used concentrate perfumes for very special occasions 30 years ago. Today eau de parfum and eau de toilette varieties, as well as concentrates, are splashed on every day by many women. The smell of flowers, or exotic and heady fragrances is one way some women project sexiness and confidence. This is clever marketing from the perfume houses, and has unfortunate consequences for those allergic to strong fragrances. Remember that no-one needs a lot of perfume during the day. In the evening, when the mood is more conducive to romance you may use the fragrances more. Scent signalling will occur naturally anyway, perfume or no perfume.

As is the case with their primate cousins, women have a different vaginal smell when they are ovulating than when they are not. Some women worry they don't smell clean, sweet or feminine enough at all times and have succumbed to the use of vaginal sprays. This is confusing for males and confusing for the body. Men instinctively like, and are aroused by, the variety of genital smells. So keep clean and let that be sufficient perfume in the genital area.

Men, please consider the aroma of your body too. Be clean. Use aftershave lotions and colognes if you want but keep in mind that less is more. Don't splash on aftershave. It is as much a turn-off as women overdoing the perfume spray. And please use deodorant, and make sure you change your shirt and underwear every day.

SCENT SIGNALLING IS POWERFUL, EROTIC, INEXPLICABLE AND POSITIVE

When a survey of sex appeal was carried out in 200 different cultures, it was discovered that clean skin was the single most important feature. It is a powerful erotic signal for our species. Scent signalling is powerful, erotic, inexplicable and positive.

Smooth skin

Smooth skin is another interesting factor to consider with skin and sex appeal. Traditionally, men and women have appreciated the difference between their skin textures. Women's skin is smoother and much less hairy than men's. Vive la difference! Running hands over exposed skin is an early signal of liking. Feeling the smooth skin or the hairy skin is a socially acceptable step in the direction of seduction. Smooth skin feels softest to the touch. Men love women's smooth silky skin. Many women enjoy stroking a man's hand, beard or face and appreciating the mix of hairs and smooth skin, strength and softness.

A current fad is the shaved head on men. What does it say at a subconscious level? It is blatantly sexual, phallic, confident and aggressive. There seem to be three groups of men engaging in this historically unusual behaviour only made possible by the advent of the electric shaver:

THE SHAVED HEAD ON MEN IS BLATANTLY SEXUAL, PHALLIC, CONFIDENT AND AGGRESSIVE

- Those who are losing their hair and see total baldness as an easier road. These men are aged from the late 20s through to 50s. It takes confidence to handle the attention and remarks directed towards their newly naked head.
- Young, aggressive sportsmen who are not necessarily losing their hair but are members of a team wishing to instil fear in the opposition. This tactic may work well since the shaved head is an unashamedly confident 'in your face' gesture.
- Young men who want to look confident, be free of society's traditional values, who desire to conform to a rebellious society and so opt for the easy care and inexpensive, or macho, look. The result is the shortest haircut imaginable with a soft fuzzy feel to it as it grows out. The message is aggression and raw energy.

Is the shaved head sexy? To some women yes, to others, no. It is certainly touchable and these men must have lots of appreciative hands run over their head. Touching a head, as we have seen, is one sign of intimacy. The positive aspect of having a shaved head is that it takes courage. The negative? It takes a hat or beanie in winter to keep warm.

Touching behaviour

Each of us has a **body contact quotient** for the amount and type of touching we require. Touching and cuddling provide security, protection, comfort, love and contentment. Research has also found that people with high body contact requirements are comfortable with their sexuality. They like to eat and talk and express their feelings easily – including their sexual feelings. Psychiatrist Dr Marc Hollender in his questionnaire and paper 'The Wish to be Held' mentioned in the book *Nonverbal*

Communication, suggests there are a small number of women with extremely high body contact scores resembling 'an addiction'. These women tend to be very insecure and are often involved in affair after affair because they find sex to be a highly efficient way to have their body contact needs met. As one woman explained 'I require hugs, and in exchange give sex; however, I want to stress often all I really am seeking is for a man to touch me.'

> **TOUCHING AND CUDDLING PROVIDE SECURITY, PROTECTION, COMFORT, LOVE AND CONTENTMENT**

It has been suggested by many women we interviewed, that it is very common from time to time for them to have sex because of the before, during and after body touching involved. Women require intimacy, with physical and emotional intensity, and being held is a sure way to achieve it.

> **WOMEN REQUIRE INTIMACY, WITH PHYSICAL AND EMOTIONAL INTENSITY, AND BEING HELD IS A SURE WAY TO ACHIEVE IT**

Most men also enjoy touching and being touched. The major difference between men and women here is the smaller number of 'cuddling addicts' as Hollender referred to them in the test sample of men compared to women. 'Men can acknowledge their longing to be held, but its intensity either does not reach the height attained by some women or, if it does, it is not reported.'

Touching and affectionate body contact are necessities for humans. Without touch we shrivel. Body contact needs express the 'like factor' we feel towards others. Reach out and touch. You will break down barriers, build rapport, feel good, and if done appropriately and gently, your friend will enjoy the experience.

Begin with the areas around the elbow and the wrist. Never begin with areas too close to the breasts or genitals.

WITHOUT TOUCH WE SHRIVEL

The colour and biology of sex

As you approach sexual intimacy both biological and colour changes occur. Blood begins to infuse the skin because of the increase in sexual desire making the skin become, to a lesser or greater degree, pink or red. With arousal blood flows from the deeper areas of the body to the surface areas. The softer areas of the body become engorged and enlarged. With this rush of blood we feel warm and there is heightened sensitivity over the entire body. At this point we are so aware of the lightest touch. Make sure it is a light touch you give your partner. Being heavy handed is inappropriate overkill.

For some people, the flushing is very pronounced. It is a bright measles-like reddening most commonly seen in women. It begins on the skin over the stomach and upper abdomen, spreads to the upper part of the breasts, then the upper chest, then to the sides and middle region of the breasts, and finally the undersides of the breasts. Often the face and neck are also coloured as Desmond Morris points out in *The Human Animal* and his earlier book, *The Naked Ape*.

This arousal and infusion of blood changes nipples as well. They become erect for both sexes. For women, nipples may lengthen by up to one centimetre and the diameter of the nipple increases by as much as half a centimetre. The areola region around the nipple also deepens in colour for women but not for men. Women's breasts become firmer and rounder with arousal, and by the time orgasm is reached the breasts of the average woman have increased in size by up to 25 per cent.

WOMEN'S BREASTS BECOME FIRMER AND ROUNDER WITH AROUSAL

Arteries pump blood so quickly to the surface with increased arousal that the veins have difficulty carrying it away, so the soft parts of the body including the nose and ears, swell slightly. The ears become sensitive to oral caresses, more so in some people than others. Some men and women report an almost direct line of arousal between ear lobes and genitals. Some find the softest blowing, sucking and licking of their ears the strongest arousal mechanism. Others say stimulating the nipple and swollen breasts lightly is what they need. Everybody has some part of their body, including the now hardened penis, that cries out to be touched. For you and your partner it is important to identify just what it is. For many it will be more than one source of arousal. All those softer areas are now engorged with blood. Slowly, so as not to hurt, touch, massage, stroke some of them and notice the response.

SOME MEN AND WOMEN REPORT AN ALMOST DIRECT LINE OF AROUSAL BETWEEN EAR LOBES AND GENITALS

The lips also become engorged with blood. They become redder, swollen and more protuberant than at any other time. You probably haven't had time to notice this. Be gentle with your touches and kissing of all the soft tissue areas of the body. This is a time when you can damage if you are too heavy-handed or kiss very forcefully.

The genitals are changing dramatically as arousal continues. The clitoris becomes erect, the labia enlarges – swollen and bright red. The penis becomes swollen with blood until it is engorged and erect.

THE GENITALS ARE CHANGING DRAMATICALLY AS AROUSAL CONTINUES

Not only are organs and tissues swelling and changing colour with sexual arousal, at the same time blood pressure, pulse and breathing rates increase. The heart beats twice as fast as orgasm approaches. Blood pressure doubles and for many men and women breathing becomes increasingly noisy and difficult. Some sound as though they are running a race as they speed towards climax.

HOT DURING AROUSAL AND HOT AND SWEATY AFTERWARDS!

With ejaculation and orgasm, all the physiological changes reverse rapidly with one exception. Most humans sweat a little or a lot after orgasm. This film of sweat develops on the back, the thighs, the upper chest, the palms of the hand and the soles of the feet. Hot during arousal and hot and sweaty afterwards!

Orgasm itself varies in intensity and frequency from person to person and couple to couple. Most people agree it is one of life's greatest pleasures because at the moment of climax you are absolutely and intensely self-indulgent and self-focused despite the fact that moments before you were emotionally and physically involved with your partner.

One interesting and very unusual phenomenon is seeing **colour at orgasm**. Some people experience an awareness of colour during the build-up to orgasm, while a few actually see colour at the time of orgasm. Those who have experienced this phenomenon, described it as 'magical', 'mind blowing', 'amazing', 'exciting', 'the feeling and effects stayed with me for days. I walked around in a dream-like state.' The colours they see range from exploding deep blue–purple patterns, to fireworks of yellow and orange, to streaks of blue, pink and white, to exploding white-silver trails of light, to minute star-sprayed firecracker-like yellow to pure light. One woman reported not only the colours but also a taste of sweetness each time she experienced these wonderful orgasms. Only a handful of people we spoke to have had this experience and almost all, only once in their lifetime. It was a very memorable experience of love for all of them.

ONE WOMAN REPORTED NOT ONLY THE COLOURS BUT ALSO A TASTE OF SWEETNESS EACH TIME SHE EXPERIENCED THESE WONDERFUL ORGASMS

With or without colour, orgasm brings release, feelings of absolute pleasure, sometimes absolute love and certainly deeper intimacy. Most of us are so busy being aroused and reaching a sexual peak we never consider the colours, behaviours and biology of sexuality. Why should we? It happens without any input from us, except the acceptance that sensuality, passion and loving are desirable. From one culture to another around the globe, the sequence of seduction is very similar. From one culture to another the visual, vocal, scent signalling, smooth skin differences and touching behaviours are very similar. From one culture to another the biology of sex is identical.

From one culture to another, seduction is instigated by the same sensual triggers.

SECTION three

bedroom behaviours

Everything in your bedroom tells a story about the intimate aspects of your life.

CHAPTER 5

up close and colourful

...colour in the bedroom

When it comes to absolute intimacy, whether shared or alone, there is one room which expresses your personality, the dreams for your romantic life, your level of contentment as well as your fantasies. It is your bedroom. The way you decorate your bedroom, the way you make the bed, the overall tidiness or messiness of the room, how clean and fragrant it is, how much time you like to spend in it when you are not asleep, whether you enjoy leaving the door open or closed, the colours and style of the room and the accessories, and the colour and style of the clothing you wear to bed all reveal your attitude to yourself, relationships and sex. *Everything* in your bedroom tells a story about the intimate aspects of your life.

When you change the look of the bedroom you change more than its colour and style. More importantly, you change how you feel about the room, how you feel about going to bed for sleep or seduction, how calm or agitated you feel. You can also change your partner's feeling about intimacy. Do you think that the relationship is too far gone for cosmetic changes to make a difference? Perhaps. Perhaps not. What we can assure you is by understanding the subconscious

WHEN YOU CHANGE THE LOOK OF THE BEDROOM YOU CHANGE MORE THAN ITS COLOUR AND STYLE

messages hidden in your bedroom you will begin to see the path of your relationship in a new light.

When you feel the need to change aspects of your bedroom's decoration or even the style or colour of your own nightwear, your colour choices will tell you what is happening in the intimate and sexual part of your life. Note the changes, listen to your heart and by looking closely at the section on colour psychology you will see yourself and relationships in a new light. If you do what you've always done, you'll get what you've always got.

This chapter examines the effect and meaning of your choice of colour for bedrooms. An important point to keep in mind is that we all move through different colour stages in our lives because of different circumstances, emotions and relationships. None of these is 'right' or 'wrong'. They just are. In the next chapter, we identify styles of decoration. You will not only achieve visual harmony in this room of rest, love and intimacy but you will discover the authentic you.

In Chapter 7, we look at strategies which make a difference in your relationships, such as what you wear to bed and its effect on your sex life and colour remedies for the bedroom. We also suggest ways to correct any inconsistencies in colour and style.

Let's begin 'bedroom behaviours', by examining the meaning of colour in your bedroom.

Identifying your overall colour scheme

Do this quick questionnaire. Glance quickly at your bedroom. What is the *overall mood or depth of colour*? Don't get hung up on particulars. Majority impression is what we are after. Is it:

- neutral
- dark
- medium
- pastel
- bright?

IF YOU CAN'T GIVE DEFINITE NAMES OF COLOURS TO YOUR BEDROOM, YOU HAVE NEUTRAL COLOURING

Now check the following information to understand its general message about you.

When you have neutral colours predominantly
... the mood is one of security.

If you can't give definite names of colours to your bedroom, you have neutral colouring. Neutrals include beige, cream, ivory, white, grey and natural wood in, for example, flooring and furniture. Many people use some neutrals because they mix with everything. In this category we mean that everything from walls, to the floor, to the fabrics, to the furniture and the accessories are all neutral in colour.

If this is your bedroom, the psychological message is *neutrality* in your intimate life. You are probably someone who likes to play it safe and not create waves. You are not prepared to make a bold statement in the decoration of your bedroom and you are probably not prepared to make a bold statement about yourself or your sexual needs. You possibly feel very neutral about the relationship you are in.

Although neutrally coloured clothes have a classically European look, neutrally coloured bedrooms are different. They indicate the most intimate aspects of your inner self rather than the image you present to the outside world. Choosing neutrals in your bedroom can indicate you are not yet absolutely sure of yourself in terms of relationships and sex, or that there is no passion or emotion involved in your intimate life.

You prefer to play it safe, rather than taking risks, when it comes to love. Of course, there are people who are worried about choosing colours which don't coordinate or harmonise well, so neutrals become a safe choice. This fear of colour risk can show itself in a fear of displaying intimate emotion too.

Neutral can be pale, medium to dark, or a contrasting combination of dark and light. The best description of neutral is natural, with neutral colours appearing often in nature. Examples can be seen in the trunks of dead trees, the bark of most trees, and in the dried stalks and vines of other plants which have been bleached by the effect of the sun.

Key words: neutral, safe, conservative, non-involvement, non-emotional.

When you have predominantly dark colours
... the mood is sombre and controlled.

When a large amount of black is mixed into colour, dark colours are created. For example, dark blue, navy, dark green, deep red, burgundy, dark brown, deep purple, deep russet, black and charcoal. Dark colours suggest control, steadiness and conservativism in intimacy. If your bedroom is dark, you are probably a refined and dignified person who likes to be in control of all experiences in your life, including your sexual experiences. Your bedroom may be luxurious, expensive, or dramatic and stimulating, yet the atmosphere will always be subdued and controlling. If you are financially very successful in business and used to being in control, you could well choose dark colours for the bedroom. You like to have control in every area of your life.

Combining dark colours with other colours will make quite a statement. If there is no lightening effect you will have created an oppressive atmosphere. Try combining darker colours with pastels, to create a softer and less controlling feeling. Adding pale pink, for instance, to a dark blue, dark green or burgundy coloured bedroom will create a softer, more loving and nurturing environment, both for the inner self and the relationship. Many people combine beige, cream, ivory or white with dark colours as a safe way to soften the look, but all this does is tone down the controlling elements of the dark colours. It does not add the loving elements.

TRY COMBINING DARKER COLOURS WITH PASTELS, TO CREATE A SOFTER AND LESS CONTROLLING FEELING

Key words: controlling, steady, serious, subdued, conservative, dignified.

When you have predominantly medium colours
... the mood is one of confidence.

Medium or mid-tone colours fall into the colour range between light and dark. You can have medium neutrals, medium brights or just medium colours.

MEDIUM COLOURS ARE UPLIFTING WITHOUT BEING TIRING

Medium colours are uplifting without being tiring. As long as they are not too muted, they have a sense of fun and lightheartedness about them. They are not as romantic as pastels, not as overpowering as the brights, not as oppressive as the darks. They are easy to live with. They exude a warm and energising feeling to most people and they can be seen as 'cocooning', giving a bedroom a sense of security and comfort.

By choosing medium colours you are making a statement. You have not chosen to be neutral at all. You are letting your boldness show, albeit gently. It tells you and the rest of the world you are taking the middle road in your relationship. You are not playing it safe as the neutral voters do. You are more adventurous than them but not as outgoing or spontaneous as someone who chooses a bright contemporary colour.

Your sex life is probably medium too, with no extremes. You are, however, confident in the bedroom and in bed. You are not ultra-romantic, not boring or safe and not too controlled. This colour choice is often a favourite of Classics and Practicals (see Chapter 6.)

Key words: middle-of-the-road, uplifting, easy to live with, no extremes, confident.

When you have predominantly pastel colours
... the mood is tranquil and inviting.

Colours with a lot of white added are termed pastel. To be accurate, you must be able to give the colouring of your room a name beginning with 'pale' or 'light', for example pale pink, light blue, pale green, light lemon, pale lilac, pale mauve, light apricot, light peach, pale aqua or white with pastel accessories. If there is no definite colour, you have a neutral.

When you want communication in your relationship to be more open, choose

WHEN YOU WANT COMMUNICATION IN YOUR RELATIONSHIP TO BE MORE OPEN, CHOOSE PASTELS

pastels. They are full of light and more free-flowing than the controlling elements of dark colours. Want more romance as well? Choose pastels. The softness of their colouring makes them non-confronting – and very seductive. A bedroom with lots of pastel colours in walls and floor coverings as well as accessories, or white walls with neutral floors but lots of pastels in bedcovers, sheets, lamps and the pictures on the wall, is most alluring and inviting. It suggests romance, love and fantasy more than any other colour scheme. If you have chosen pastels for your bedroom, you are romantic, sensitive and looking for nurturing, love and fun in your intimate life. You will be friendly and non-threatening in your intimate experiences and will want to receive exactly what you have portrayed in your bedroom: to be treated gently, thoughtfully and with sensitivity by your partner.

Pink and peach are the most romantic pastels because they send the subconscious messages of love and communication (the psychology of colours is explained a little later). They are also very flattering against all skin tones. If you shudder at an all pink or peach bedroom, take heart. It is not necessary to have all pink or all peach to add romantic overtones. Just a small amount will do, perhaps in sheets, pillow slips, accessories or even on the walls. The room could be very very pastel or could have some stronger highlights of these colours. There will be however an identifiable amount of peach or pink in the room.

Not all pastel bedrooms have pink or peach in them. The general feeling with other pastels is one of tranquillity and composure. Some people, however feel that the use of predominantly pastel colours creates an insipid, superficial atmosphere. There is no way they want a romantic light look.

Up Close and Colourful

Key words: light, open, soft, inviting, romantic, tranquil and composed.

When you have predominantly bright colours
...the mood is fun and vital.

Bright colours are purer colours with no black and very little white added. For bedroom decoration they include bright cobalt blue, bright yellow, orange, red, hot pink, lime green, bright purple and anything else bright you can think of. Often two or even three brights may be positioned together. What does it say about you? Bright colours suggest movement, vitality, happiness, cheerfulness, youthfulness and fun. They are striking, contemporary colours which create a modern, casual look. If you have chosen bright colours for your bedroom, you are an outgoing person with a great sense of fun. Your sex life is probably spontaneous and innovative.

> **BRIGHT COLOURS SUGGEST MOVEMENT, VITALITY, HAPPINESS, CHEERFULNESS, YOUTHFULNESS AND FUN**

The negative aspect of using bright colours is that they can be overpowering and tiring in a bedroom, because they are so exhilarating. We hope you sleep well. If your day life is busy and stressful you will quickly tire of brights in your bedroom. Perhaps not at first for sex, but certainly for sleep. These colours are not romantic, but exciting and, often because of the energy expressed by them, it is only children and young adults who choose this option. For the rest of us, accents of brights can add interest to a more conservative style bedroom and create an energy and lightheartedness in our inner selves. In a holiday home, brights create freedom and energy to uplift us when we need a break from everyday stress.

Key words: vital, fun, youthful, contemporary, casual.

You've discovered the overall impression your bedroom has on mood and behaviour. Now it's time to look at what the colours actually mean.

Colour psychology

POPULAR COLOURS AND THEIR SUBCONSCIOUS AND CONSCIOUS MESSAGES

There are many variations when it comes to colours and even the names given to them. We will only look at the most popular, which will certainly give you plenty of scope to identify the meaning of the colours you have chosen. If you want to understand, for example, the meaning of cobalt blue, electric blue, baby blue or duck egg blue, read the following basic blue messages, consider your choice of brightness or paleness and make adjustments accordingly. Use this as a general guide for understanding colour in your bedroom.

Do this quick questionnaire. Glance at your bedroom once more. What is the *overall colouring*? Don't get hung up on details. Majority impression is what we are after.

What colour have you chosen for:
- the walls ....
- the ceiling ....
- the floor* ....
- the furniture ....

  * with natural timber floors and furniture decide whether the colour is closest to brown or beige.

What colour is the bedspread or doona cover, sheets and pillowslips? ....

Look at your main bedroom accessories. They add their own colour power, but are minor players.

What colours are the:
* lamps ....
* cushions ....
* paintings? ....

Now you have an overview of your predominant colour scheme. We have listed below the colour psychology of your choices. Look at our information for the predominant or major colour in your room and then check the meaning of the other colours you have used for accessories.

If your room is predominantly blue

A bedroom decorated with blues is a calm and restful oasis. When you need some peace and quiet in your life, blue is the way to go. It signifies commitment and contentment, but be careful it doesn't create boredom in your intimate life since blue can dampen the emotions and create moodiness and melancholy.

A BEDROOM DECORATED WITH BLUES IS A CALM AND RESTFUL OASIS

Dark blue is very peaceful and calming but can stultify emotions and become oppressive unless other colours are introduced to add warmth and balance. Pale blue is lighthearted and inspiring, the colour of a free spirit. For some, because of its coolness, it may indicate an amount of icy superficiality.

Your choice of blue could suggest you are trying to appear cool and confident to hide a vulnerable inner self. If you are *blue biased*, you need a partner you can trust, as loyalty and honesty are important to you. When you are in a relationship, you form a strong attachment to your partner and are deeply hurt if your trust is betrayed. Your sense of duty and responsibility often overtake your own inner desires and needs.

If your room is predominantly pink

Being a pale version of red, pink still has passion and energy in it, but not as much as red. If you have chosen a predominantly pink bedroom you wish and need to be treated with love, thoughtfulness and caring, and you will want to reciprocate those feelings. It is useful to add a touch of pink to every bedroom to awaken love, compassion, nurturing and understanding. If you *pine for pink* in your bedroom it may indicate you have a need to protect your inner self, and perhaps that you are afraid to show your own vulnerability.

> **IF YOU HAVE CHOSEN A PREDOMINANTLY PINK BEDROOM YOU WISH AND NEED TO BE TREATED WITH LOVE, THOUGHTFULNESS AND CARING**

Because pink is a feminine and intuitive colour, many men find it uncomfortable to be in a bedroom dominated by it, so be aware of this when decorating – small touches are often better when it comes to pink or red. When we discuss the styles of bedrooms you will discover that pink is typical of the Romantic.

If your room is predominantly green

If green is your preferred bedroom colour, you have created a retreat from the stresses of the external world. This is your area to retire to and be healed. *Gravitating to green* gives a sense of relaxation and rejuvenation in your bedroom, as though you are communing with nature in your own private rainforest. You have a deep longing to be loved and to belong, and relationships are very important to you and your wellbeing. Various forms of green are often used in Practical style bedrooms (see Chapter 6).

People favouring greens are pragmatic, realising the fundamental use of a bedroom is for rest and sleeping, and green is the best colour for this. If you have trouble sleeping, try having a green bedroom or at least placing some of this colour in a prominent position in the bedroom.

IF GREEN IS YOUR PREFERRED BEDROOM COLOUR, YOU HAVE CREATED A RETREAT FROM THE STRESSES OF THE EXTERNAL WORLD

If your room is predominantly peach, or apricot or orange

A bright orange bedroom would be definitely over the top and not conducive to sleeping. Instead, choose a soft peach or apricot, as these colours have some vitality without being too stimulating, and they are liked by both men and women. They are warm, inviting and stimulate communication at all levels, particularly physically.

SOFT PEACH OR APRICOT ARE WARM, INVITING AND STIMULATE COMMUNICATION AT ALL LEVELS, PARTICULARLY PHYSICALLY

If you *pulsate for peach* and *have an appetite for apricot*, you are an optimistic and socially outgoing person who loves being around other people. You are fun-loving and adventurous, but can sometimes appear to others to be fickle and insincere. Deep down you may have an inferiority complex which you are working on overcoming with your gregarious and uplifting personality.

These very pastel forms of orange are often used in Romantic style bedrooms or sometimes in the Town and Country style, where they are combined with textured natural fabrics.

If your room is predominantly yellow

Yellow is an intense colour and suggests fun, happiness, pleasure and some intellectual stimulation. A bedroom decorated with a large amount of yellow indicates a relationship based on a more mental form of communication, rather than being based on a purely physical or emotional relationship.

With yellow predominant, especially a bold yellow, you are likely to be a perfectionist who is very critical of yourself as well as others. The inner you loves a challenge and change is always welcome, otherwise you feel easily bored. When you *yearn for yellow* you are broad-minded and rarely have any inhibitions, although there may be more talk than action in the bedroom. You may actually spend more time analysing and talking about your sex life than actually participating in it. You are an inquisitive person who asks a lot of questions.

> **YELLOW IS AN INTENSE COLOUR AND SUGGESTS FUN, HAPPINESS, PLEASURE AND SOME INTELLECTUAL STIMULATION**

Bright or intense yellow is best not used in large amounts in a bedroom as it can create anxiety and keep the mind too active, both of which are not conducive to restful sleep. It's best to choose a very pastel version such as cream, buttercup, pale lemon, or pale golden yellow, or use it in a very small quantity. Alternatively, complement strong yellow with deep blue, deep green or deep purple to reduce its stimulating impact.

Bright yellow is often combined with other primary colours in a Contemporary style bedroom and usually only chosen by young adults or children who seem better able to handle the energy of this colour.

If your room is predominantly purple, or lilac, or mauve

Purple and violet are powerful colours which people seem to either love or hate. It would be difficult even for the most ardent fans to live in a house full of purple and violet. To many they are spiritually uplifting colours, while to others they are depressing. Deep purple should be used sparingly by anyone prone to depression since it can inhibit the emotions in susceptible people.

Those who have chosen colours from the purple and violet spectrum, including mauve, lavender and lilac, have an imaginative bedroom where dreams and fantasy reign. You are a creative person who likes to be considered different and individual. You are also poised, refined and dignified with a set of strong values with which you are comfortable, even though they may be unconventional. Perhaps you are inclined to live in a fantasy world to hide the uglier side of the real world. Those with a penchant for purple and for the lighter tints of the purple family are often sensitive and intuitive. This can sometimes lead to moodiness if you spend too much time in your bedroom alone. You need to be treated with love and dignity in your intimate life as you continually yearn for emotional security.

> **DEEP PURPLE SHOULD BE USED SPARINGLY BY ANYONE PRONE TO DEPRESSION**

> **PURPLE ITSELF NEEDS ANOTHER COLOUR WITH IT, SUCH AS WHITE OR CREAM, OR A SOFT GREEN TO KEEP IT EMOTIONALLY BALANCED**

So if you are *partial to purple*, lilac, mauve or pale violet are certainly better choices than bright purple or dark violet for a bedroom. They are softer and more romantic. Purple itself needs another colour with it, such as white or cream, or a soft green to keep it emotionally balanced. It is better for you to use in small amounts as an accent rather than decorating an entire bedroom with purple, unless you absolutely adore it and don't share your bedroom with anyone else.

If your room is predominantly turquoise

Turquoise, a greenish blue, is a very calming colour to use in your bedroom. It creates a friendly atmosphere which nurtures communication from the heart and balances the emotions. If you find yourself *turning to turquoise* you are looking for balance in all areas of your life and wish to develop an inner calm to help you deal with stress. Sharing and togetherness is important to you and you feel you need to create an emotional relationship with someone before you can have a physical relationship with that person. Once this emotional connection has been established, you do not like to be rushed in lovemaking.

TURQUOISE NURTURES COMMUNICATION FROM THE HEART AND BALANCES THE EMOTIONS

Because you want balance, you are often not spontaneous in your actions. You need to think things through. Sometimes you find it hard to make decisions in your emotional life, and yet in other areas of your life you can be very decisive, making you the best person to have around in a crisis.

Turquoise combines well with greens, blues and oranges, as well as the colours of love – deep pink and magenta. It is important to use a small amount of another colour with turquoise to prevent over-emotionalism in a bedroom. Any colour from the red spectrum will be effective, such as red, pink or magenta. It is often used in Contemporary style bedrooms, teamed with other bright colours.

If your room is predominantly a medium blue-green

Blue-green in all its variations (some of the names given include jade and teal) is a positive prestigious colour suggesting success and confidence. All aspects of image are important to you, so for example, you will be very well groomed. Blue-green is calming, without depressing the emotions.

BLUE-GREEN IS A POSITIVE PRESTIGIOUS COLOUR SUGGESTING SUCCESS AND CONFIDENCE

If you have chosen this colour for your bedroom you are a compassionate and confident person who likes to stand out from the crowd a little. You are sexually self-confident, yet individual in your intimate pursuits. *Brimming with blue-green* is positive. You can choose mid to deep blue-green to express yourself. The best colours to combine with it are pink, lemon, pale turquoise, cream and lilac. Using small amounts of red as an accent with blue-green is also a confident expression of who you are.

If your room is predominantly red

Red is the colour of energy and action and the use of large quantities is usually too overpowering in a bedroom. Red is the colour of sexual passion and excitement. If your partner redecorates your bedroom in red, it certainly indicates that he or she wants a lot more passion, excitement and sex from the relationship. This would be a very obvious indication of needs. A more subtle introduction of red as a part of the redecoration of a bedroom indicates that more passion and excitement in the relationship is a desirable outcome.

RED IS THE COLOUR OF SEXUAL PASSION AND EXCITEMENT

If you have chosen a lot of red in your bedroom, you are an energetic and exciting person to be with, although your partner may find it difficult to keep up with you. You love being the centre of attention and may have an inflated ego. Routine is not a part of your life as you move from one venture to another, looking for the next exciting and stimulating adventure. You tend to be impulsive, competitive and aggressive and yearn for excitement in all life has to offer and as fast as possible. *Relishing red*, you like to live life in the fast lane, especially in bed!

Red is best used as an accent in any decorating scheme, as it is too action-oriented to create a calm and relaxing sleeping environment.

If your room is predominantly brown

If you have chosen brown for your bedroom, you may be trying to create a safe cocoon within which to withdraw from the pressures of daily life. Brown gives a feeling of comfort and security to many people. It is also a colour preferred by a lot of very down-to-earth people who like the stability and strength of material security. These people are reliable, steady and serious-minded.

BROWN IS SERIOUSLY SENSIBLE

On the other hand it can also be a sign of discontent. Brown is deep. Brown is not fun. Brown is seriously sensible. If you're *browsing with brown* think hard whether the relationship is too static. Predominantly brown in a bedroom could cause boredom in a long-term relationship. Add some pink to the room and this will infuse more loving energy without taking away from the comfort and security of the brown.

If your room is predominantly beige

Beige is a neutral chosen by many because it is safe. It is a less intense form of brown, creating a quiet confidence and sophistication from which to build a base. If your room is predominantly beige, you have decided to be very neutral in this most intimate of rooms. You don't like to make waves. The overall effect can change slightly depending on the base colour within the beige, such as pinky beige, blue beige or yellow beige. If you are *beckoning beige* you are very careful to keep a calm atmosphere in the bedroom with very little passion or excitement to stir the emotions.

> IF YOUR ROOM IS PREDOMINANTLY BEIGE, YOU HAVE DECIDED TO BE VERY NEUTRAL IN THIS MOST INTIMATE OF ROOMS.

If your room is predominantly cream

Cream is another neutral colour which is safe in home decoration. Because it contains more yellow in its base colour, it is more uplifting than beige. In all other aspects it has a similar effect to beige in that it is safe and calm. If you're *crazy for cream*, you understand it creates a soft and warm bedroom environment, slightly more intimate than white and as a neutral, stands you in good stead. Cream suggests you want your intimate life to proceed smoothly.

> CREAM CREATES A SOFT AND WARM BEDROOM ENVIRONMENT

If your room is predominantly white or soft white

Many people have embraced a major white look at different times in their lives. It can occur when seeking a clean start after a major emotional change, perhaps after a marriage breakup, or at the end of a relationship, or after physical or emotional upheaval. White helps during times of stress and creates a clean slate from which to make a new start.

White helps during times of stress and creates a clean slate from which to make a new start

If you have chosen a predominantly white bedroom, fairness and balance will be important to you. You will be cautious in your intimate life, and tend to be a perfectionist who is often over-critical of yourself and others. Self-sufficiency will be a trait you have developed. Being the symbol of peace, white creates a feeling of tranquillity and hope for the future.

With a *wistful white* decor, you risk creating an atmosphere of sterility. If this is not what you want, add some colour to the room such as pale pink or pale green to stimulate the emotions and senses.

If the room is predominantly black

Black as the predominant colour in a bedroom can indicate a person who is trying to create a seductive, mysterious and sophisticated retreat. You are intent on luring your prey! It always suggests control and power over others. Black can also indicate someone who wishes to hide from the outside world, or perhaps someone who is going through an unhappy period in their life with a great deal of inner emotional turmoil.

The black bedroom may also frighen off a prospective lover

If this is your choice of colour for a bedroom, it may be that you associate black with sophistication, seduction and sexiness, as in the black negligee, or you may be a secretive person who is prone to depression. It is wise to keep black, in large amounts, to clothing. It is a very intimidating colour wherever and whenever it is used. Combined with a lot of red, the black bedroom would indicate an aggressive person who wants to control and dominate. Unfortunately it may also frighen off a prospective lover.

Are you *blinded by black?* The predominantly black bedroom is usually associated with a Dramatic style bedroom. It is really inappropriate to have an almost all black bedroom. It is the negation of all colour, so black should be used as an accent and combined with other strong colours or white to balance its energies. Love would not be a factor in this bedroom. Domination would be.

If your room is predominantly grey

Grey is a colour used by those who look at life with too much realism and caution. In a bedroom it indicates someone who is cautious yet persistent in their sexual life. A colour of emotional control, it can indicate a person who is hiding true feelings since it is so neutral and colourless. To lessen the neutrality, if you are *grabbing for grey*, team it, depending on the base tone in the grey, with pink, blue, yellow, green, red, peach or apricot to enliven and enhance positive energy in your bedroom.

GREY INDICATES SOMEONE WHO IS CAUTIOUS YET PERSISTENT IN THEIR SEXUAL LIFE

Creating Balance with Colour

Decorating with colour can be a daunting experience for many people. This explains why neutral colours are used so often in homes. They are safe. Do try some other colours now you know the meanings. Experiment with accessories or new bed linen. Understanding how to use colours effectively is fun. You will also feel very different about your bedroom and what goes on in it when you have a little courage.

Using complementary colours in your bedroom

The use of complementary colours can do more than enhance the look of a room. They also create emotional balance. The predominant use of any colour has a psychological impact, so adding a complementary colour to the scheme can balance the psychological effect of the main colour. This is very appealing visually and many of you already intuitively do this.

The use of complementary colours can create emotional balance

The basic complementary colours are:

RED	COMPLEMENTARY	GREEN
ORANGE	COMPLEMENTARY	BLUE
YELLOW	COMPLEMENTARY	PURPLE

Think carefully before combining colours. Consider the intensity of each colour. When you place complementary colours next to each other, they intensify one another. While in some settings this works, it can also be overpowering, and softening the intensity of one of the colours may create a more appealing combination. Play around with accessories, samples of fabric or even paper to see the effect of using complementary colours in your bedroom. Think how well red and green go together in Christmas decorations. Unless the balance of each colour is carefully addressed in a bedroom, this may be overwhelming. However, choosing a lighter green with some ivory or cream, then adding accents of red can create an eye-catching combination.

Purple and yellow in their purest form may be too overpowering for most of us. Predominantly yellow in a bedroom may make you over-critical and analytical. Predominantly purple in a bedroom may take you into the escapist fantasy realms. What to do? In the yellow room, add touches of purple to balance the mental energies of yellow. In the purple room, add touches of yellow to balance the imagination.

Orange and blue constitute a strong combination, probably too strong for a bedroom, yet soft peach or apricot, with accents of dark or bright blue is stunning. The truth about colour is that it is an individual choice. What one person likes, another abhors. It is absolutely personal and shows the emotional connection to colour.

THE TRUTH ABOUT COLOUR IS THAT IT IS AN INDIVIDUAL CHOICE

Other combinations which work well together are:

TURQUOISE — WITH RED, OR PINK, OR MAGENTA, OR LEMON

YELLOW — WITH DARK BLUE, OR ELECTRIC BLUE OR DEEP GREEN

PALE BLUE — WITH DEEP PINK OR MAGENTA

MEDIUM TO DARK GREEN — WITH PEACH, APRICOT OR GOLD

With all other types of colour schemes, such as harmonious and triadic, the ensuing mix of colours will also create emotional balance.

BALANCING COLOUR IN THE BEDROOM

To assist you in choosing combination of colours, follow this easy guide. Surprisingly, perhaps, it is important to use colour in unequal amounts to create a balanced effect. Fifty-fifty will not work. The following percentages are approximate. You don't need to measure. Your eye will guide you to calculate the percentage of certain colours in a room. Practise on all the rooms in your home.

If using two colours, have them in the following proportions:

> 70% AND 30%
> 75% AND 25%
> 80% AND 20%

If using three colours, use the following proportions:

> 70% TO 20% TO 10%
> 75% TO 20% TO 5%
> 80% TO 15 % TO 5%

The addition of any more colours would then need to be in very minute amounts for the colour scheme to have coherence. It is also better not to decorate with one colour only, as the psychological impact can have a negative effect on the emotions. You can add a touch of a contrasting or complementary colour to balance the emotional effect of the monochromatic colour simply by using accessories or even plants.

If you feel confident in using and combining colour, play with it, experiment, have fun. Create your unique look based on intuition.

Creating your own oasis

Is your bedroom a refuge from the hectic outside world, a place where you can escape from the children? Is it a place you love to go to recharge your batteries? If it isn't, perhaps you need to look at your own needs, and create a space there which is inspiring and relaxing for you to retire to whenever you feel the need. Make it an oasis of peace, pleasure and calm for yourself or with your partner.

> **MAKE IT AN OASIS OF PEACE, PLEASURE AND CALM FOR YOURSELF OR WITH YOUR PARTNER**

If you have negative feelings about your bedroom, look closely at your life and examine the intimate and sexual aspects of it. Are there issues in this area that you need to sort out, or past events you need to discard, or repressed emotions you need to deal with? Believe it or not, redecorating the bedroom, a little or a lot, will bring these issues to a head and help to clear the energy. This is healthy.

If you cannot change the bedroom at least change the colour of the towels in your ensuite bathroom leading from the bedroom. If you don't have an ensuite, then look at your family bathroom. The bathroom is an emotional extension of you, so even a move as small as differently coloured towels can influence your mood.

Making even small colour changes in your bedroom can indicate your changing emotional needs. If you find yourself needing to put white flowers or white sheets into the bedroom you are really seeking new beginnings in your life, or within your current relationship. Pink sheets may indicate that you are in need of some tender loving care. Adding green touches may suggest a need for relaxation and rejuvenation. If an overactive sex life is leaving you exhausted, add some green to the room to create more balance – maybe a plant. If blue is involved in your changes, you may be looking to create a calming respite from a hectic lifestyle.

You have identified the colour choice you have made in your bedroom and its psychological subconscious impact, so what next? You can:
* acknowledge and muse on where you are up to in your sexual life
* change a few items of colour to change your relationships
* do nothing and enjoy what you have
* decide to explore your heart and needs and discuss your unhappiness with your partner
* if you live alone, create the bedroom you'd love to have, one which will give you great pleasure and satisfaction

> We all move through different colour stages in our lives because of different circumstances, emotions and relationships. None of these is 'right' or 'wrong'.
> They just are.

CHAPTER 6

intimate design

... how bedroom style plays its part

The following questionnaire will help you to identify the decoration **style** you have chosen for your rendezvous with sensuality, passion, emotion, affection, rest and sleep. After all, your preferred choices give you and a partner, a bird's eye view of the way you make sense of the world.

A bedroom questionnaire

1. Please tick your answers. Is your bedroom basically:
   (a) frilly and detailed
   (b) softly romantic with curves
   (c) classic with clean lines and angles
   (d) tailored and neat
   (e) practical and basic
   (f) comfortable and textured
   (g) dramatically different in colour or design
   (h) filled with the influence of Italy, Mexico or another recognisable country
   (i) cottagey or rustic
   (j) a creative mix of furniture and styles from anywhere and everywhere
   (k) modern with clean lines
   (l) themed and dream-like
   (m) simple, neat and comfortable

(n) bold with shiny surfaces
(o) like entering and being immersed in a different country
(p) bright, colourful with few accessories
(q) like a trip to another place and time
(r) cluttered with unusually arranged memorabilia

Identifying answers: (a) romantic; (b) romantic; (c) classic; (d) classic; (e) practical; (f) town and country; (g) dramatic; (h) ethnic; (i) town and country; (j) creative; (k) contemporary; (l) fantasy; (m) practical; (n) dramatic; (o) ethnic; (p) contemporary; (q) fantasy; (r) creative.

2. Tick the other decorative items you have in the room
    (a) pictures
    (b) paintings
    (c) photos
    (d) small accessories
    (e) something humorous
    (f) other furniture
    (g) lamps
    (h) bedside tables/drawers
    (i) mirror
    (j) what is on the wall above your head as you lie in bed?

3. What styles in your accessories can you identify according to the suggestions in question 1?

4. Look around and decide:
    (a) Is my bedroom comfortable?
    (b) Is it really how I want it to be?

5. Is the overall appearance:
    (a) boring

(b) too dramatic
(c) too neutral
(d) too anything else?

6. Does the look of my bedroom relate to how I feel about sex?

7. Does the look of my bedroom relate to the state of my sex life at the moment?

What your answers reveal

Your answers to the last questions will open your eyes to your relationship and challenge you too. The style of decoration in your bedroom may relate a little or a lot to the overall decoration, or to the architectural style of your home. Old houses and apartments lend themselves to an old world look. If your home has Victorian era detail, it is appropriate to repeat some of those details with the interior. You may, for example, be influenced by Romantic and/or Classic styles since that time period in social history reflected them strongly. If your home is very modern, then you could decorate with a more Contemporary feel than in another home.

Having pointed out the merits of consistency with the history of your home and your decoration, we also want to suggest you don't have to follow the architectural style at all. We've seen lots of homes with the outward appearance of a particular style but the moment the front door is opened, wow! The interior is so different. The key is to be consistent whether you are being sensitive to the architecture or whether you completely change it. Also be authentic about who you are – you don't have to adopt someone else's style.

BE AUTHENTIC ABOUT WHO YOU ARE – YOU DON'T HAVE TO ADOPT SOMEONE ELSE'S STYLE

Now is the time to create a feel, a style that is just you. If you surround yourself with a neutral, bland style, you tend to be neutral and bland in your behaviours, just to keep the peace and avoid risks. Don't you think it is time to become the authentic you?

THE COLOUR AND STYLE OF THE BEDROOM LAY BARE THE REAL PERSON

By discovering your bedroom decorating style you will have a better understanding of yourself and others. Most importantly when it comes to sexual relations, you will have an inkling of what a partner expects at both conscious and subconscious levels. The colour and style of the bedroom lay bare the real person, more so than any other room in your home. It indicates how you like to be treated.

How do you check out the style of a potential partner if you are single? The rest of the home gives you some ideas. By asking what pieces of furniture he or she really likes you will begin your understanding, but the bedroom says it all. Take a quick look at it if you can, as you walk past it on the way to another room. That peek will give you an overall impression.

Once you spend the first sexual occasion in your new lover's bedroom, appraise it with an educated eye. That's when you have time to do a sweeping stocktake of the bedroom decorating style as you relax in bed. You have already appraised the loving style. Keep in mind that we are all on our most romantic best behaviour the first time we go to bed with a new partner so first impressions aren't necessarily accurate.

ONCE YOU SPEND THE FIRST SEXUAL OCCASION IN YOUR NEW LOVER'S BEDROOM, APPRAISE IT WITH AN EDUCATED EYE

Let's slow down a moment. This book is not just about enhancing relationships. It is, more importantly, about understanding *you* in your relationships, in romance and in sexual intimacy. Taking time to digest the styles listed, and relating them to your bedroom decor, is a wonderful way to come close to yourself today. Then you can be guided if and when you want to make changes.

To help you understand the style you have created in your bedroom, we have identified nine categories. Any styles you feel we haven't listed are really part of one of the nine. Remember too, you may have a combination of styles in your bedroom. You have to identify the major ones. Deep down, the styles you have chosen are an accurate reflection of who you are or who you were when you decorated the bedroom.

To help you give a name to your preferred styles, imagine describing your room to a friend who has never seen it. Choose a word or phrase most aptly describing the sense of your bedroom. Perhaps you would say romantic, perhaps bold and dramatic, perhaps practical, perhaps well-ordered and always neat, perhaps cottagey. The word you choose also describes you.

Most people have chosen a combination of two (or even more) styles because:
- you like a mix of styles – it suits your personality
- you have to share the bedroom with a partner whose style is different
- you don't know about style – you have collected pieces of bedroom furniture from all over and they seem to work
- as long as you have somewhere to sleep, who cares about style?

- your authentic bedroom style represents the personality you express with clothing and that is frequently a combination as well.

You've thought of the words to describe your bedroom by now. So read the descriptions below carefully to understand yourself and the big picture. Find a style or two which leap off the page at you. You will also be able to identify the predominant style in the bedrooms of others. You might find it easier to decide what's *not* your style. Perhaps your path will be to use a process of elimination.

BE YOURSELF, MAGNIFIED AND MAXIMISED

Remember that no one style is better than another. Be yourself, magnified and maximised. Being true to who you are and expressing it with colour and style in this intimate haven will reveal many truths to you and your partner. Have fun with it.

If your bedroom doesn't inspire you and you are unsure of the style you really like, buy or borrow lots of magazines and see if you can find a style that you'd love to create. Follow our descriptions of each style to give you a base from which to create a unified bedroom style in harmony with your inner self.

Nine readily identifiable styles of intimate design

Remember most people are combinations of decorating styles. For example you may be a Classic–Town and Country mix. Read both styles in detail and look closely at your bedroom. When you notice things that aren't either of these styles, choose from one of the styles that is yours as a replacement. The room will seem to come together for you then.

CLASSIC

The Classic bedroom is elegant, dignified and controlled, as is the person who chooses it. It is a tailored look that is visually balanced, with no extremes in its presentation.

The Classic preference can be seen in the choice of tailored bedspreads rather than the soft comfort of a doona.

> **THE CLASSIC BEDROOM IS ELEGANT, DIGNIFIED AND CONTROLLED**

The way the bed is made tells you a lot about the Classic style too. Everything is straight, level, and immaculately even and neat. Pillows and cushions are placed formally and symmetrically. Piped edging on bedspreads and cushions is typical. There is a classy and neat finish to all decorative embellishments.

Fabrics are of good quality and either plain or with traditional patterns. These patterns are often geometric rather than curved, although traditional florals are sometimes used. Classics always have quality drapes, usually pleated, and usually with a pelmet or draped fabric across the top to give an immaculate finish to the window. Curtains are often elegantly tied back with well made and tailored corded tassels. Frills are not a feature. They are too romantic for a Classic. Wallpaper is often used and is always traditional or understated in pattern and colour.

Colours in fabrics are usually neutrals or muted medium to deep tones of blue, green, dusty pink or burgundy. Sometimes an all-over monochrome look in soft white or ivory is chosen for fabrics, with dark furniture breaking up the colour scheme.

Furniture is either darker classic timbers such as mahogany, rosewood or walnut, or lighter timbers such as western cedar and oak. Its styling is traditional if not antique.

The Classic bedroom is classy and traditional with medium size patterns and medium size accessories. Symmetry is important so you won't find any unusual abstract patterns or artwork on display. Some may say Classic is boring. Classics would not. They insist subtle, classy and good quality are the essence of good decorating.

SYMMETRY IS IMPORTANT SO YOU WON'T FIND ANY UNUSUAL ABSTRACT PATTERNS OR ARTWORK ON DISPLAY

Classic mixes well with other styles, probably because of its balanced and simple styling. As a Classic you could find yourself adding dramatic touches to create the Classic–Dramatic style, or perhaps creating a softer look to give the mix of Classic–Romantic. A popular combination is Classic–Town and Country where texture and country, plant or animal motifs become part of the theme. A certain elegance will be apparent when Classic is combined with another style.

The bedroom of a Classic, whether he/she mixes other styles with it, will always be a visually balanced room, with no jarring elements to upset its symmetry.

CLASSIC ACCESSORIES have smooth, simple and elegant lines. Lampshades are plain, neutral or pastel in colour, or sometimes in a darker colour to blend with the room or to match the bedspread. The shade may be plain or pleated. The lamp base is simple and elegant, not textured, sometimes the smooth wooden antique look, or a traditional cylindrical shape, or ornate antique style brass. Cushions on the bed match the bedspread or certainly harmonise with it and are very structured and formal. Often there will be no cushions at all. Paintings are realistic scenes, flowers, animals, or portraits.

They are elegant artworks rather than contemporary abstracts. Picture frames are antique, silver, or timber with clean, elegant lines. It is very common to find framed family photos in a Classic's bedroom.

Mirrors are timber, either antique or smooth dark timber. Crystal dressing table sets and matching brush and comb sets are typical traditional Classic accessories. Ornaments in the form of collectibles, placed perfectly in groups on the dressing table or chest of drawers are also typical.

There are two distinct types of Classic bedroom:

1. The traditional style, which uses darker coloured antique furniture, such as rosewood and mahogany. Softly draped chintz type fabrics with traditional (and somewhat old world) designs based on roses are commonly used. Piping and tassels may feature. Traditional is the most detailed and tailored look in Classic style bedrooms.

2. The modern style which uses lighter coloured classically styled furniture which never dates. These pieces are not extreme and probably can't be given a date. They follow well-accepted style lines. In this modern look, a few antique heirloom pieces are sometimes added because they are quality Classic items. Fabrics still drape well, although they may not necessarily be as tailored as the traditional style. Bedspreads are immaculately smooth and everything has a neat and tidy finish. Sometimes a doona may be used, but it is very smooth, with a pleated rather than gathered valance. It is a well-groomed look though softer and slightly more relaxed than the traditional style.

The female Classic bedroom has either tailored floral fabrics or quality plain fabrics which fall in soft lines. Colours are most likely neutrals with the barest touch of colour to them, or traditional muted blue, green, maroon or dusty pink. It may have some romantic elements to it as well, as the Classic woman often likes to soften the image of the elegant classic style when it comes to bedroom decoration. The room is always neat and tidy and often has soft flowers in traditional vases. The Classic woman is at all times a well-groomed woman.

The male Classic bedroom has the best quality plain fabrics, or geometric patterns such as some tartans, herringbone or other angled lines, usually in fairly subdued, more masculine colours of dark blue, dark green or burgundy, with a neutral contrast of beige. This bedroom has a very elegant, serious look, rather than being soft and inviting. It is always neat and tidy and the bed is always well made.

You can read the **personality of the Classic person** by looking closely at the bedroom. Here is a conservative, stylish, elegant person who may appear aloof but who opens up and is softer with friends. The Classic person has a well-balanced body shape, with no extremes in facial appearance: straight nose, medium-sized mouth and usually oval face. The Classic is of average height and weight. The hair is always well groomed and not too long. If there is long hair, it is frequently tied back. Even the way they walk and sit tells you this is a controlled person. The posture is good, the sitting and placement of the legs, slightly formal. Actor Pierce Brosnan and the late Princess Grace of Monaco are good examples of Classic personalities.

> **THE CLASSIC PERSON IS A CONSERVATIVE, STYLISH, ELEGANT PERSON**

This conscious awareness of themselves as even, balanced and physically average appears in their home environment too. Balance is a key. Nothing too extreme, please, we are Classic. Everything has to be neat and tidy inside and outside the house. Control of the environment is important. Let's have quality lives, quality relationships and quality control, is their credo.

Sexual responses will be mainly traditional; occasionally something unusual in bed will occur, but modesty is a component of the Classic personality, although every Classic has a little (sometimes very tiny) piece of Dramatic trying to get out.

Bravo! Let the Dramatic emerge. You can still have a neat and tidy bedroom, but add a bold touch with colour or unusual accessories. For example, a striking sculpture or a large painting add drama to a traditional Classic bedroom without changing the tailored elegant effect which Classics love.

Key words: controlled, tailored, elegant, visually balanced, neutral or subdued colours of traditional blue, green, maroon, burgundy, dusty pink, or neutrals.

TOWN AND COUNTRY

The Town and Country bedroom is a casual, relaxed and friendly style. Its main focus is physical comfort and texture. With its design based on casual country style living, both curves and angles are used, often together. It is an inviting and comfortable, yet sturdy country look which also works well in the city.

TEXTURE IS THE MOST OBVIOUS FEATURE OF A TOWN AND COUNTRY BEDROOM

Texture is the most obvious feature of a Town and Country bedroom, with both visual and tactile texture being apparent in fabrics and furniture. The smooth polished clean lines of Classic are not for Town and Country. They prefer the sturdy, chunky, well-worn or distressed look of country style timber furniture. The bed is often wooden with bed ends.

This style of bedroom has either a soft and inviting doona, or a patchwork bedspread. Often, because of the style of bed chosen, there is no need for a valance. It is not a tailored look at all. Sheets and pillowslips are cotton fabric in plain natural colours, cottage prints or gingham checks. Many large soft pillows are on the bed as they add to the creation of a comfortable and inviting atmosphere. Symmetry in placement of pillows or accessories is avoided since being neat and tidy is not of prime importance to a Town and Country.

Colours used in furniture are natural and neutral tones of off-white, cream or beige, or light- to medium-coloured timbers are popular. Fabrics are in natural or neutral colours or medium-toned colours similar to those which appear in cottage prints. Texture is almost always a feature on any plain fabrics used for curtains, bedcovers and seats.

The Town and Country style is a great mix of city conveniences teamed with the feel and comfort of the country. The best of both worlds. These people choose medium to large scale furnishings and accessories and often mix patterns because in nature that happens anyway. They make texture on chairs, bed covers, photo frames, picture frames, carpet or timber floors, light fittings, furniture, fabrics and dried flowers an essential element, even if they are unaware of it.

ACCESSORIES IN A TOWN AND COUNTRY style bedroom often create a cluttered, but at closer examination, a fascinating look. This gives the feeling of comfort, cosiness and warmth to the occupants. Town and country people love to accessorise their bedrooms with quirky, country style, distressed objects such as old tin chests and old suitcases. The list of accessories includes such items such as wicker furniture and wicker baskets, wash stands, basins and jugs, patchwork items, interesting country style wooden animals, shells, candlesticks, wreaths and flower garlands, dried flowers, fresh flowers, and handmade craft items. There is often a sense of humour and whimsy present and a little clutter.

There are three basic Town and Country decorating styles. Perhaps yours is definitely one of these or perhaps a combination of one with another style.

1. The cottage Town and Country style bedroom is cosy and comfortable with cottage print cotton fabrics, or gingham checks or a patchwork bedspread. A cluttered and busy look is often achieved with many handmade craft items decorating the walls and top of chests of drawers and dressing tables. The old and the new mix well here and the look of distressed timber and country cottage items is preferred in this style bedroom.

2. The Town and Country style emphasises all that is natural: natural colouring, natural-coloured timber furniture and textured natural fabrics. It will always have a doona rather than a bedspread, with many large, soft pillows on the bed to create a cosy, comfortable and welcoming atmosphere. Because they are very tactile people, the fresh feeling of crisp cotton against their skin is very stimulating to the natural Town and Country type. Fresh and natural is of utmost importance to this type of Town and Country.

3. The French provincial Town and Country style is charming with an informal elegance and a touch of romantic. It uses light European timbers for its larger pieces of furniture. The curved lines of armoires and side pieces enhance the casual grace and elegance of this style. Cords and tassels are often used, as is heavy white lace for curtains, bedspreads, cushions and lampshades.

The female Town and Country bedroom may have the natural, casual, textured look or it may have the country cottage look of cotton fabrics with small floral prints such as the Laura Ashley prints, the French provincial look or the natural look. Comfort is of prime importance. She likes natural, light- to medium-coloured, stained or painted timber furniture and a mix of textures. Bedroom colours will range from neutrals to pastels to mid colours. Cane and wicker often appear in the bedroom. Several comfortable cushions on the bed complete an inviting picture. However the cushions will not be absolutely perfectly placed the way a Classic would neatly arrange bed accessories. Several comfortable cushions on the bed complete an inviting picture.

COMFORT IS OF PRIME IMPORTANCE

A male Town and Country bedroom will have lots of texture in the fabrics with an emphasis on natural colours of cream, white, beige or brown. There will be a lot of natural, light coloured timber furniture. It will be a welcoming and comfortable room inviting you to enfold yourself in the security and cosiness of its soft and comfortable style. The bed will be made but to a Classic it looks messy and untidy. Visual perfection is not a priority to them.

How does this type of decorating reflect the **personality of the Town and Country** man and woman? Natural finishes for me, they say. No polyester or plastic – let me be in touch with nature. Let me reflect on the lives of the early pioneers and their simple, functional and recycled furnishings. I can adapt all that to my city lifestyle. I can do a little creating of my own by, for example, rubbing back a table, or sifting through the discarded and pre-loved furniture in the many wonderful antique or old wares shops.

The out-and-out Town and Country person loves touching the textures. They run their hands over old furniture or fabrics and love the tactile sensation. And they wear textures themselves with style. No plain smooth fabrics – they are into comfort and easy style with textured cotton, linen, wool, silk.

> **THE TOWN AND COUNTRY PERSON LOVES TOUCHING THE TEXTURES**

When recognising a Town and Country person away from their home environment, notice the height (often taller than average), the build (angular rather than curved) and the angles in the face. These tell you that comfort in clothing and shoes is very important to them. The overall impression is friendly and approachable. They laugh a lot. Sarah, the Duchess of York, Robert Redford and Clint Eastwood are good examples of Town and Country types.

With this understanding of the pure Town and Country man and woman, you can begin to identify the personality that flows so easily with their decorating style. It is friendly, welcoming, unpretentious, take me as you find me, and enjoy the bounty of nature. Here is a person who wants to feel comfortable and shows it.

In bed? Lots of pillows please because that's generous and if they are feathered pillows, they are so comfortable. What about sex? Yes please. That is so natural, but it must be sensual and involve touching and more touching and appreciating the lovely smell of the fresh sheets, and the yummy natural smell of you.

Key words: cosy, casual, homely, comfortable, textured and natural country style.

ROMANTIC

The Romantic style is based on sensuality and curves, frills and lace. It is a soft and cosy, perhaps even cluttered look where everything is in sensual harmony. Feminine and inviting is how most men see it. This bedroom can seem over the top to some, while to others it is heavenly. More than any other style it is blatantly soft and sensual, which can be interpreted as a sexual invitation. Wait to be invited in! While they may appear to be soft and vulnerable, Romantics do not like to be taken advantage of and are really quite in charge of their intimate life.

THE ROMANTIC LOOK IS A SOMEWHAT SOPHISTICATED AND GLAMOROUS LOOK WHERE SMOOTHNESS AND SENSUALITY, RATHER THAN TEXTURE, PREDOMINATE ON THE SURFACE FINISH OF FABRICS AND FURNISHINGS

The Romantic look is a somewhat sophisticated and glamorous look where smoothness and sensuality, rather than texture, predominate on the surface finish of fabrics and furnishings. Fabrics are sheer, or net, or decorated with a floral design, or maybe even in a luxury fabric such as velvet. Sometimes a mosquito net floats above the bed. Curtains, usually gathered, drape softly, sometimes into a pool on the floor. The curtains are voluptuous and full, never skimpy. Sheets and bed linen are soft and luxurious, sometimes in satin. Doonas are used more than formal bedspreads since they create a softer, more cosy and inviting look. Whatever the bedcover, it is sensual and inviting, sometimes in lace such as broderie anglaise, sometimes in a floral design and nearly always has a frill around the doona cover. When a valance is used, it is gathered quite generously.

Frills and lace always feature somewhere in the Romantic bedroom, even if it is just on the doona or on the pillows or cushions on the bed. And there are extra pillows and cushions. These are not only for comfort but also as a display of generosity. Romantics are generous in all aspects of their lives. They are not restrained when it comes to true love and romance.

ROMANTICS ARE GENEROUS IN ALL ASPECTS OF THEIR LIVES

Curves, rather than angles, predominate in the Romantic bedroom. Furniture has curved and rounded lines. The bed may be a four-poster, decorated with soft netting, lace or frills, or an ornate brass bed with curves on it, or simply one with a curved bedhead. Other furniture has curved lines or may be softly draped with a fabric cloth or a detailed table runner. Sometimes sets of drawers, the bedhead or bedside tables have intricate carvings on them. Curved decorative touches in the form of painted finishes such as floral stencils on walls and furniture, perhaps cherubs somewhere or decoupaged items are sometimes evident. The overall look is quite busy and cluttered, both in quantity and design.

Colours are either delicate, soft or understated, in white, pinks, apricot or peach, or in a mixture of pastels or in the deeper more opulent colours of burgundy or maroon. Romantics love to create a soft, cosy and cuddly retreat filled with their sentimental collectibles and they love fresh flowers in the room. There is a little of the Romantic in everybody so touches of it may appear in the other styles as well.

While the Romantic bedroom seems very feminine, there is also a male Romantic look which has some of the elements of this style. Romantic men are often the charming Romeos we meet.

ACCESSORIES in a Romantic bedroom are soft, lacy, frilled or old world. Lamps have ornate carved bases or are softly rounded or made of antique glass. The shades are frilled, fringed or lacy, with a softly gathered look. Cushions are soft and lacy or frilled. Paintings have a very romantic feel to them, often with buxom women as the main theme, or cherubs and angels. Frames are carved, detailed or ornate, but definitely not plain. Photo frames and mirrors are ornate silver or brass, or carved wood or hand painted with ornate floral designs. Ornaments are almost always mementos or collectibles of some kind and they will have a nostalgia about them. This is the one style which is highly decorative and usually quite cluttered, creating a sensual warmth and cosiness.

There are three basic Romantic decorating styles:

1. The antique Victorian Romantic has lots of lace and frills, cosiness, comfort and clutter. Soft and filmy fabrics feature here, sometimes with a lacy mosquito net. These bedrooms are usually decorated in all white fabric and lace combined with medium to dark antique furniture, with lace runners or doilies, or lace tablecloths covering them. Fringes and bows with trailing ribbons may be a part of the decoration as well.

Occasionally, some pastels are used. Four-poster beds in decorative wrought iron, brass or ornate antique polished timber are usual. The total effect is soft, lacy and curvy, with no harsh lines. Pillows are soft and plentiful with lacy or frilly covers. Ornaments and mementos are plentiful and cover every conceivable surface.

2. The modern Romantic style has voluptuous softness as the main feature. Fabrics will be soft and delicate or opulent and may have floral or softly blended geometric designs, or they may be plain and pastel. The colours used are soft pastels of pink, blue, green, ivory, peach or white, or combinations of these colours. Furniture will be of medium- or light-coloured timber, or it may be painted timber, often with decorative stencils on it. There may be round tables with frilled tablecloths, and family photos displayed with other mementos on the tables, as well as roses or other romantic flowers. There is a certain amount of fantasy involved in this type of romantic bedroom, as these Romantics often like to escape from the harshness and inconsistencies of everyday reality. Where better to do it than in the intimacy of the bedroom?

3. The subtle Romantic style is a toned down version of the modern style. It is still very seductive, yet not overly lacy or frilly. Abstract curves in furniture and fabric designs will feature and colours may be stronger. Paintings or sculptures of nudes will often appear in accessories. This bedroom will be dramatically romantic and sensual rather than softly romantic and sensual. This will often be the choice of the Romantic male.

The **female Romantic** bedroom is one of the above styles using lace, or frills, or soft floral fabric, or sheer curtain fabric or a combination of all. It will be a very feminine room, but one that is loved by men even though they would not decorate in such a manner themselves.

We usually don't think of a male bedroom as being Romantic, but a **male Romantic** is usually a more dramatic romantic. This is where you see the black mosquito net, which creates a seductive and mysterious atmosphere of allure. It invites and lures you into his web of intrigue. Abstract curved lines are another indication of a male Romantic, although these curves are often more dramatic than the female Romantic bedroom. Colours are stronger and the room could also have an old world, antique look to it, with a lot of medium to dark timber furniture contrasting with softly draped fabrics, with influences from the classic style. It has more furniture and accessories in it than other male bedrooms.

So what about the **personality of a typical Romantic**? As we discussed earlier, body types and personalities mirror bedroom styles. This room is you at your most intimate even if you share it with your partner. Imagine yourself as a complete Romantic lying resplendent on soft sheer fabric. Imagine yourself tantalised by satin, lace, or perfumed pillows and a partner wearing the sexiest next to nothing, white or pastel underwear. The Romantic can show you all these pleasures. Their bedrooms invite you to indulge. So be indulged and expect it from them all the time in their behaviour.

ROMANTICS SEE THEMSELVES AS VULNERABLE

Romantics see themselves as the most vulnerable, the easiest to bruise, even the saddest of all people. They are more needy than most and need to be indulged. They are flirtatious. They want you, and they think and say it often. If they are more reserved they will think it more than verbalise their feelings. Expect a lot of romantic, sensual talking between the sheets. And on the telephone. They know how to use their voice, their eyes and their bodies. It's not just the sexual you they want, its also being around the physical you. They want to hold hands. They stroke you. They fight for the limelight. When two Romantics get together, that, as a Romantic woman friend told us, 'is wonderful but dreadful. He wants to be centre stage but I do too. I saw his bedroom and felt so envious. That's how I wanted mine to look.'

They want sensuality and romance to be the most important thing in your life as it is in theirs. Lead with your heart. They certainly will. A Romantic is very choosy about where they have sex. If you are thinking of a hotel, for instance, check it out very carefully and be prepared for rejection and complaints if romance, cleanliness and sensuality isn't expressed in the room. And definitely forget the camping holiday.

The Romantic is of medium height, usually, but not always, has softness and roundness in their facial appearance. This could be represented in full cheeks, dimpled chin, roundish or heart shaped face, full lips and big eyes. Romantics more than other styles like lustre, soft and subtle, in their clothing – a silk blouse, stockings with a subtle sheen, a suit or tie with a slight sheen. Both men and women also have curvy bodies. Let's explain that.

Many Romantic women are curvy, from their curly (sometimes permed) or wavy lustrous longish hair to their full bodies. Some will be full busted and full hipped. Some, just full hipped and thighed. Some will be petite and still have curves. They are the finer boned version of the feminine goddess. Even for them however, the lashes are long and curvy (perhaps with the help of mascara) and the lips full. It is difficult to find a Romantic woman who does not wear perfume and make-up, especially eye make-up. The eyes express so much intimacy after all. Detail becomes them, from their detailed jewellery of small to medium size to their detailed clothing.

Men also have Romantic curves. Muscles, average height and wide shoulders lead down to a definite waist; (well that's when they were in their twenties and thirties) and a great backside – curved and shown off in well-fitting trousers. That is the focal point for Romantics of both genders. They do love to show off their bodies in well-fitting clothes. The men look suave and choose European-style clothing.

Romantic men also have full lips, long eye lashes and wavy or curly hair. (Some Romantics do have straight hair but they wish it had more wave.) Some have a dimple in the chin. You see how their physical appearance is full of natural curves? There is nothing stiff about the way they move. Both the male and female Romantics walk and move in a very sensual way. They sway. They glide smoothly. They also love to choose clothing which is great to touch. Silky, soft and sensual is for them.

Elvis Presley, Leonardo DiCaprio, Dolly Parton and Oprah Winfrey are examples of Romantics.

In bed? Romance and more romance please. Let's be sexy and intriguing with clothing. Touch me sensually and lightly. Stroke me. Let's not reveal everything too quickly. Let's not rush. Let's have mood lighting, or candles, and soft music. What passion and sensuality is in store!

Key words (female): soft, sensual, feminine, curvy, frills, lace, floral, filmy, pink, pastel colours or white, cluttered, highly decorative, glamorous, softly sophisticated.

Key words (male): curved lines, stronger mid-tone colours, abstract curved designs, cluttered, cosy and cuddly, sensual, glamour with dramatic or classic overtones.

DRAMATIC STYLE

A Dramatic style bedroom is strong and bold and has extremes in everything. It is sophisticated, innovative and flamboyant, and a little intimidating to others who are not so dramatic. These people are bold, confident and in control in all aspects of their lives. They like to be the centre of attention and their bedrooms reflect that too, as does their sex life.

> **A DRAMATIC STYLE BEDROOM IS SOPHISTICATED, INNOVATIVE AND FLAMBOYANT**

Furniture has sharp and well-defined lines. It may be matte finish or very shiny. It is probably black or chrome. The bed is plain and simple in line, maybe in black wrought iron, or black timber. There are no decorative features on it. Strong abstract and geometric designs, large abstract florals or strong contrasting plain colours in fabric are a feature. Designs and patterns in fabrics are large and dominant and make a definite statement. Wallpaper, if used, is bold, sometimes in deep red, black, gold or black and white.

There is usually a strong contrast in the colours used. Walls are often painted in very dark colours, with a light contrast used for the rest of the furnishings. Red or black or gold, and sometimes all three, usually appear somewhere in the decor. A black mosquito net can tell you they are Dramatic (with a touch of Romantic). There is no use of frills or softly draping fabrics. Windows often have dramatic looking blinds or black venetians, rather than curtains.

Dramatics are the ones with the animal print bedroom. Not the tiny animal print look, but the big look. Why pussyfoot around if you have Dramatic tendencies? They are passionate and energetic people, sometimes larger than life, and it shows in any decorative elements they incorporate in their decor. Sexual, bold and direct is the style; it is impossible to ignore a Dramatic.

Accessories in a **Dramatic** bedroom are bold. Lamps are unusual and individual. Lampshades are strong and bold, clean lined and always make a statement. Paintings are abstract and large, with perhaps one large piece dominating the walls. Photos are not usually displayed, but if they are they will be in unusual and striking frames. Mirrors are large art pieces in themselves, probably in striking colours or flamboyant shiny gold. Blatant sexuality may be evident in statues and other art work.

There are two types of Dramatic bedrooms:

1. The extreme Dramatic makes a statement with every item in the room. This can be intimidating and only the most Dramatic of people could live with it for any length of time. Relaxation and sleeping don't come easily in a bedroom like this.

2. The subtle Dramatic, which is a toned down version, has a few items in the room making a statement, but overall it is not as intimidating. You can recognise the subtle type because of the use of red or black somewhere in the colour scheme

without them dominating. If not red or black, there is strong contrast in the colour combination.

The **female Dramatic** bedroom has much creative flair to it. Animal prints, or bold bright combinations of colours such as black, red and gold are used. There is always something eye-catching in the room, whether it be in the design on the doona, an object on display, or the colour combination itself. The female bedroom is often more subtle than the male Dramatic's bedroom, though it will still have a very confident air. Something shiny, burnished, highly polished or with a shimmer could well be a feature too. Lacy black underwear or lingerie could be on display, with feather boas adding another Dramatic touch.

The female Dramatic bedroom could be intimidating to a male suitor. He may be wondering if whips or bondage are part of the activities! Keep the door to your bedroom closed until the new man gets to know you. Then your bedroom may well excite him.

The **male Dramatic** bedroom has strong contrasting colours, such as black, red and white, or animal prints which 'bring out the animal in them'. The lines are usually angular and geometric. The room will be extreme in colour and design. These men are confident, bold and dominant. They like to be noticed and are often exhibitionists. This will be evident in their sexual style as well.

What is **the personality of a Dramatic**? Bold, outspoken, self-assured, decisive and sometimes aloof. Anyone who is prepared to decorate a bedroom boldly with colours, designs and styles others shy away from, has to be confident. The bedroom suits them. The Dramatic man or woman has a distinct and dramatic appearance. They are usually taller than average with long arms and legs. A Dramatic's body and face is somewhat angular. There are very few curves on the body. That's why they are attracted to angles in design too. Their hair will be the latest fashion or even extreme and severe in cut. It will always be controlled. No curves here, angles appeal. These hair styles look appropriate on Dramatic men and women. Their clothing styles are the latest, the boldest and often European styling.

Nothing ordinary. Nothing small and simple. It just doesn't work. Forget lots of detail. Clean sweeping lines are in. And shine. Not just lustre. Shine and gloss.

Examples of Dramatic personality types include Cher, Jim Carrey, Naomi Campbell and David Bowie.

Which brings us to the bedroom behaviour of Dramatics. What would you expect? When the bedroom is set up for drama, expect it. It isn't soap opera stuff based on emotions. This is loud, clear, decisive, perhaps unusual sexual and sensual behaviour. 'You want what?' you say. Nothing too ordinary. The Dramatic woman loves to wear black or red lacy lingerie and suspender belts with black stockings.

Foreplay? Yes. 'But let's not pussyfoot around. Let's get on with the sex. Let's try different positions. Let's spice up this relationship. Let me show you how.' Yet underpinning all this is a sense of formality and authority. The Dramatic is confident in bed and out of it. They know it, do it, enjoy it, and move on to the next fascinating episode.

Key words: contrasting elements, strong colours such as black, red and gold, extreme, bold, confident and dominant, flamboyant and sophisticated.

PRACTICAL

Comfort, utility and easy care are the key points for the Practical bedroom. These are the down-to-earth, functional people in our world. They're the ones who are quite happy to accept all the bits and pieces offered to them by relatives and friends, even though the pieces may not match anything else. Being practical, they always find a way to incorporate them into their homes. Practicals are collectors and often hoarders, who don't like to throw out something which may be of use in the future. They are the bargain hunters of the universe. As material security is important to Practicals, hoarding possessions gives a feeling of security and comfort.

> **COMFORT, UTILITY AND EASY CARE ARE THE KEY POINTS FOR THE PRACTICAL BEDROOM**

The Practical bedroom is always comfortable though not particularly soft and cosy. It is not always immaculately neat and tidy, but always clean, well kept and ordered in its appearance. Simple and uncomplicated, with any unnecessary items removed is how Practicals like it.

Furniture is basic and only in the room if there is a purpose for it. A bed, wardrobe, chest of drawers and maybe bedside tables are all that are necessary. Sometimes even the bedside tables are deemed unnecessary. Furniture is usually of natural timber, since that doesn't require any maintenance except dusting and an occasional polish.

Fabrics are patterned, in small to medium size designs, so they don't show dirt and stains, and they are wash-and-wear so there's no ironing. Frills and lace are minimal, if at all, because they need careful laundering. A bedspread is often preferred to a doona as it is a nuisance having to remove the doona cover all the time for washing. On the other hand, some Practicals prefer a doona because it is easier to make the bed with it than with blankets and a bedspread.

Curtains are sometimes used because Practicals do like their privacy. They are not the exhibitionists of this world and don't relish the idea that someone could see into their bedroom. Male Practicals often have only a blind on the window.

Only essential accessories are in evidence in this style bedroom, as they all need to be dusted. Intricate ornaments are put away in a cupboard to be viewed during nostalgic family occasions.

Colours chosen in a Practical bedroom are usually variations of those found in nature, such as green, blue, brown, gold and autumn shades. White or very pastel colours are not considered appropriate because they are not practical enough. These orderly people put time and effort into coordinating their decorating scheme so everything will match. It is never a hotchpotch of mismatched items. Price and value for money are the prime reasons they choose particular furnishing items. They do like good quality, just not the most expensive.

Some young people start out as Practicals, as accepting hand-me-downs in furniture is the only way they can set up their own homes with their limited finances. Many find their own style when they can afford to buy what they really like, while others remain Practicals for life. Since Practicals are very easy-going people, they won't fight you if you want to add some softer touches to the bedroom. In fact, although they may not admit it, deep down they will probably love it. Just don't go overboard with the changes.

Accessories **in a Practical bedroom** are usually very functional, minimalist and necessary. They include lamps which are easy to clean, without any decorative elements to catch dust, and a book they may be reading on the bedside table or the floor. A notebook is often beside the bed to write down ideas and thoughts which may come to them during the night and prevent them from sleeping. They are prolific list writers. Family photos may be displayed because family is very important to Practicals.

The **female Practical** bedroom has medium-toned fabrics, which are practical and easy care, with designs which don't show marks or stains. Plain-coloured fabrics are rarely used, and then only as top sheets and pillowslips. There are no feminine touches of frills or lace as the female Practical isn't particularly overtly feminine. (Perhaps she could consider using a draped curtain or some softness in the bedcover design and choose colours to soften the look.) The Practical woman relates well to men and is often the sporty, outdoor type.

The **male Practical** bedroom is not too different from the female room as this is a style which is neither feminine nor masculine. It may have fewer items in the room, as most Practical style men do not see the necessity for bedside tables and lamps. Often there are items of furniture handed down from well-meaning relatives and the Practical man would never throw out something which still has a use.

The **personality of a Practical** is simple, uncomplicated and pragmatic. They are the salt of the earth, 'wholesome' as a friend described them and probably the easiest people to talk to. They are above all friendly, down-to-earth and unpretentious. They are refreshingly authentic. They are the natural-looking people you come across; they can be short or tall, are usually sturdy in appearance, not sophisticated in their outlook nor glamorous in their appearance – but certainly real.

THE PERSONALITY OF A PRACTICAL IS SIMPLE, UNCOMPLICATED AND PRAGMATIC

They usually enjoy sport and outdoor activities. Some of the women were tomboys in their youth. That's the life they loved and still hanker for and you can see them in their jeans, slacks and T-shirts or polo shirts most of the time. Casual suits them best in appearance and behaviour. Often their hair is straight and easy to look after. Practicals ask the hairdresser for 'a good cut'. Some of the men like having a beard or moustache. They will not be slaves to fashion and grooming. Often they have no idea and no interest in what's in fashion for clothes or decoration. They do not overly decorate themselves or their homes. They wear lots of natural fabrics. Neither women nor men like wearing clothes that are tight since comfort is very important. For women, stockings are only occasionally worn because they are uncomfortable and not natural. Very little jewellery and make-up is used for the same reason. In fact they tend to decorate their bodies with the same colours they decorate their bedrooms.

They have colour and pattern harmony in the bedroom but nothing unnecessary and none of the sophistication that appeals to a Classic. Being practical and functional is what they ask of their clothing, their furniture, their crockery, their car and their friends. What wonderfully warm friends they are.

Good examples of Practicals are Dawn Fraser, Dick Smith, Tom Cruise and Ellen Degeneres.

The bedroom behaviour of Practicals is simple and comfortable. Very little subterfuge here. They do like romance and will sometimes team it with a degree of athleticism. Nothing particularly beguiling for them but it's absolutely genuine. Talking before and in bed is necessary too. And when it is over, 'we've got to get a good night's sleep so we can function well tomorrow'.

Key words: simple, plain, uncomplicated, useful, practical, easy care and no unnecessary decoration.

CONTEMPORARY

The Contemporary style has sharp, clean and angular or curved lines, yet with a relaxed holiday feel. Contemporary is a modern individual style using unusual and strong combinations of colour, where form and design is of utmost important. It is chic, trendy and light-hearted, with a minimal use of decorative elements.

Furniture is smooth and streamlined, often in an unusual shape, either angular or curved.

CONTEMPORARY IS CHIC, TRENDY AND LIGHT HEARTED

Stereos, televisions and books are stored in purpose-built cabinets so they don't dominate the room. Light coloured timbers, painted timber, chrome and wrought iron are often used. The 1950s style of furniture is one favourite of a Contemporary.

Texture is not a feature. A doona is mostly used, although sometimes a bedspread with simple and uncomplicated styling is preferred. The look is smooth, not soft and fluffy. Fabrics are simple and plain, with solid colours or abstract geometric patterns, or with bold checks or large spots. Small prints or florals do not feature in a Contemporary bedroom. Rather than curtains, Contemporaries prefer bare windows or just a blind for privacy. If curtains are used they are simple and plain.

Colours are bright and make an individual statement, in blues, turquoises, pinks, oranges, yellows and reds. Sometimes the theme is black and white, maybe with an accent of one of the bright colours. In others there could be a geometric print using combinations of several brights. The overall look is usually light, bright and open.

Minimal decoration is the choice of Contemporaries, so one or two large, individual art pieces or sculptures on display at any one time is usually the norm. Contemporary is not cluttered or busy-looking. It is a sparse and simple form of decoration with furnishings which make their own individual statement. Although similar in some aspects to the Dramatic style, the Contemporary look is more casual, light-hearted and fun.

ACCESSORIES in a Contemporary bedroom are few; the design of the furniture and its placement create the interest. Lamps are simple, possibly geometric and angular in shape, or unusually curved. Lights attached to the wall are preferred. Nothing appears in these bedrooms unless it is there as part of the design of the room. There are no accidents. Placement for line, colour and design is all important. Mirrors also have simple frames and photos are not on display unless in an unusual frame which fits with the whole design of the room. Sometimes Contemporary style bedrooms have one or more large pot plants as part of the decor.

There are two types of bedrooms in this style:

1. The minimalist style, which has only the most necessary items in it. This is a visually pleasing room, rather than a tactile or sensual bedroom. It often has polished floorboards and blinds on the windows. Walls are plain. There is no

wallpaper, no floor rugs, no curtains, no soft lampshades, and no upholstered furniture. Tubular steel, leather and canvas are often used. Colour is kept to a minimum and often used in a dramatic way, with no more than two colours used. Yellow with dark blue is often used, as is black and white or red and white (but not red and black since this is Dramatic). This is often a male-decorated bedroom and is popular with architects and designers who prefer to see the elements of the design rather than having unnecessary items around as distractions.

2. The modern Contemporary bedroom is stylishly individual and unusual in design and colour. It is softer than the minimalist style, yet still more severe than other styles. Colours are strong and bright, with unusual colour combinations creating a stunning individual look, for example, bright combinations of turquoise, yellow, pink, orange or green. This style suggests a casual holiday atmosphere and is usually chosen by younger people and those who are very creative or confident and outgoing. Holiday homes are often decorated in this style, as the colours create a vibrant, happy, fun and easy-care atmosphere and pleasurable holiday memories.

The **female Contemporary** bedroom tends to be the modern style of contemporary bedroom rather than the minimalist style. Fabric designs are abstract and colourful, with combinations of bright blue, pink, turquoise, red, orange and yellow. Multi-coloured geometric patterned doonas are combined with matching curtains, plain curtains or wooden slat blinds. Polished wooden floors are common, sometimes with a rug beside the bed as something soft to put feet on in the mornings.

The **male Contemporary** bedroom is often the minimalist style with more angular lines and no soft decorative elements. Men tend to prefer plain strong-coloured doonas as opposed to the multi-coloured variety. Men also don't see the need for unnecessary items of furniture or decoration. Polished floorboards are common in the male Contemporary bedroom. Colour is secondary to the design lines of the furniture.

The personality of the Contemporary is similar to the Dramatic: clear, direct yet more relaxed and colourful. Expect contemporary social behaviours to be reflected in terms of rights, sharing of tasks and emotional and sexual expectations. What does a Contemporary person look like? Contemporary. They prefer European designers, or unusually talented local designers. They can display lots of colours put together carefully or adore basic black. A little shine appeals too.

They are usually slim and striking in their appearance, with more angles in the body design than curves and the clothing choices will have angled simplicity which has its own built-in sophistication. An example of a Contemporary was Diana, Princess of Wales.

What will not go down well in the sexual relationship is the mundane or the ordinary. Contemporary people are seemingly sophisticated and almost always very stressed. They work hard and play hard. They lead very full lives. When it comes to sexuality they could well be like the rest of us. 'Sex? Yes please and a lovely night's sleep. I am exhausted.'

Key words: sharp, clean, modern, trendy, angular lines, minimal colour or bright multicolour, no fussiness, minimal furniture, minimal decoration, relaxed casual holiday feel.

CREATIVE

The Creative bedroom is individual, unique, artistic and non-conformist. It is an eclectic mix of furniture and furnishings brought together with creative flair using unusual colour combinations and accessories. Colour is often the unifying element tying everything in the room together. This style is absolutely individual and so diverse that we cannot give a specific template for it. However you will recognise it when you see it as the style of the free spirit. In fact, Creatives would hate to think they fitted into any of these styles at all, even the Creative one. They don't like to be boxed.

> **THE CREATIVE BEDROOM IS INDIVIDUAL, UNIQUE, ARTISTIC AND NON-CONFORMIST**

There is no symmetry or uniformity and nothing will match in the bedroom. Bedside tables are often different, not only in style but usually different from each other. Lamps are unusual, and furniture is a mix of pieces acquired from other family members, second-hand stores and local markets. Usually this means it is in well-worn or distressed timber. Sometimes it is creatively hand painted.

> **COLOUR IS OFTEN THE UNIFYING ELEMENT TYING EVERYTHING IN THE ROOM TOGETHER.**

Beds have everything from doonas, to old bedspreads, to coloured and patterned fabrics covering them. They may be textured or plain. Curtains are lace, or a multi-coloured fabric or just a sheet hung creatively over a window.

Colour may be the only unifying element in the whole room. And colour there is. Bland and boring neutrals are never acceptable to a Creative. Quite often yellow is the unifying colour which appears in all the fabrics in the room. Purple is another Creative colour favourite.

Designs on fabrics are small to medium in size, with abstract geometrics being favoured. Patterned scarves and multi-coloured fabrics are often thrown over furniture or hung on a wall. There may be some items from another culture. Beading and fringes often appear on everything from lights to furniture. Cushions, large and small and in a multitude of different fabrics are found on the floor or bed. It is a somewhat cluttered look and quite untidy, but very much loved by the Creative personality.

COLOUR MAY BE THE ONLY UNIFYING ELEMENT IN THE WHOLE ROOM

Creatives are bower birds who love rummaging around at local markets to collect all sorts of unrelated items and they somehow find unique ways of combining them to create their own style. This may well look like an appalling mess to many people, but it is easy to see the owners are artistic and creative individuals.

The one thing common to all Creatives is the passion they feel for each item in the room. They often feel strong emotional ties to furniture and accessories, no matter whether they are family hand-me-downs or fascinating market finds. There is always a story to tell with every item.

Yet some Creatives have a more ordered look, with unusual art pieces dominating the room, perhaps with an abstract nude behind the bed. Collections of curios such as unusual musical instruments, may decorate other walls. Creatives always find unconventional ways to combine and display their bits and pieces.

ACCESSORIES in a **Creative** bedroom include unusual items placed together with perhaps colour (even the same colour or opposing colour) as the common factor. Textures vary and nothing is used that is mass produced, or copied from anyone else, or used in a conventional way for them. That's too predictable. One thing you can be sure of, the creative loves the bedroom and its treasures and loves to take you on a guided tour if you ask. Another constant with a Creative – the bedroom will not stay looking like that for too long. Creatives decorate the bedroom for themselves and part of the fun is to make constant change.

The **personality of the Creative** has little to do with body shape, and more to do with artistic leanings. Creatives are just that, artistic and creative. They will put together in their bedroom, their house and on their person, unusual, eclectic and sometimes way-out mixes of colour, style and adornment.

They hate to conform to society's seemingly rigid rules. They like to be individual and unique in their expression. The world is full of Creative people. You see them when you shop. Most artists and many musicians are Creative. Elton John, Jack Nicholson, Paula Yates and the character of Kramer, played by Michael Richards, in Seinfeld are excellent examples of Creative people.

So what about their behaviour in the bedroom? Because a Creative seeks different ways to give and receive pleasure, you may well be delighted by their innovative ideas. The Creatives enjoy sexual talk in bed. There could also be a certain amount of theatrics. Whatever you do, don't be a conformist yourself. Society's traditional standards don't particularly interest them.

Key words: mixture of styles, bits and pieces, spiced with colour and decoration that doesn't appeal to everyone, free and eclectic, individual, unusual and unique, non-conforming.

Fantasy

In discussing the Fantasy bedroom we are referring to an adult's bedroom, not a child's room. This style will be a little 'out of this world', an escape from reality. The form of the escape depends on the type of fantasy involved. The person with this style of bedroom is obsessive, creative and individual, who uses their bedroom and their intimate life to escape from the practical and everyday issues of life. They have very high and unrealistic ideals and are disenchanted with their own reality so the intimate world of their bedroom gives them a chance to pretend for a while. For a brief moment the romance of another time or another life, whether it be in the past or the future, becomes their reality.

> FOR A BRIEF MOMENT THE ROMANCE OF ANOTHER TIME OR ANOTHER LIFE, WHETHER IT BE IN THE PAST OR THE FUTURE, BECOMES THEIR REALITY

With each type of Fantasy style, there is an underlying base of one of the other styles. The ethereal type is often a Romantic or a Creative, while the futuristic type is often based on Contemporary or Dramatic. The impossible ideal type may be any one of the other styles. With maturity or a change in their circumstances such as marriage, the Fantasy person reverts to their basic style.

As each type of fantasy is quite different, it is not possible to give general guidelines to identify this style, except to say the bedroom decor reflects the fantasy and is totally recognisable when you see it.

There are three basic types of Fantasy style:

1. The ethereal fairytale style of the past has lots of white and light pastel colours, in particular pale mauve, pink and blue.

Fabrics are sheer and voluminous and draped everywhere. Decorative elements include fairies, cherubs, dragons, stars, moons and clouds, all in excess. This bedroom becomes a world within a world, indicative of either the immature adult seeking to find the little girl in herself, or a highly imaginative person trying to escape from the ugliness of the real world.

2. The futuristic style of the idealistic space traveller is a more stylised decorating style, with elements relating to outer space such as robots and space ships or futuristic planes. It is the world of *Star Wars*. All elements to this design have streamlined, clean and clinical lines with much silver or chrome, grey and white used. Sometimes touches of red, black or yellow are also evident. Again, this is a person, usually male, trying to escape from their present reality, this time into a world of the future.

3. The impossible ideal style is the world of Hollywood movie stars, of famous entertainers and of wealth and fame. The person who has this style of bedroom imagines that the world of everyone else is much better than his or her own and that money and fame solve all problems. Of course they only see the romantic side of this other style of living and this is what they try to create in their intimate life. The interest in the lives of celebrities, whether living or dead, by the fantasy seeker is totally obsessive and unrealistic, and that is how they live their lives. To most of us, this is immature and unimaginable behaviour – we don't understand or want to understand for that matter. It may be interpreted by many as too cult-like.

The **female Fantasy** bedroom usually involves the first type of fantasy bedroom. It has sheer white and very pastel fabrics, creating a filmy misty atmosphere in which to retreat from the ugliness of the real world.

The **male Fantasy bedroom** comes from the future or science fiction. It has chrome, silver, grey or white in it and decorative items may be suggestive of outer space and the future. The *Star Wars* theme is popular mainly with teenage boys, although some young adult males do seem to be fans.

The **personality of a Fantasy seeker** is a certainly creative one who is obsessively preoccupied with unrealistic goals. There is no one body style. This style has developed because the person has become obsessed with fantasy or is escaping from the ugliness or disappointments of reality. We cannot give a living example of the Fantasy personality since it is often a private world they enter in their bedroom.

In bed you will be impressed with the role-playing and unusual demands. Join in for a ride to another world. In time you may well be annoyed with the tunnel vision of this dreamer unless you also share the fantasy.

Key words: creative, individual, 'out of this world', an escape from reality, obsessive.

ETHNIC

We include this bedroom style because it is recognisable yet in harmony with every other style so far discussed. It is based on a style related to a particular country or culture. The bedroom and often the entire home could reflect a passion for Japan, Mexico, Bali, Spain, Greece or any other culture. There is authenticity in the representation of the cultural style. This is not a bedroom merely created from decorating magazines. This is a style loved by the inhabitant because either this is their ethnic roots or that they have become so enamoured with another culture they wish to recreate it at home.

THERE IS AUTHENTICITY WHEN A PERSON REFLECTS THE ETHNIC STYLE. THERE IS RESPECT FOR ALL ASPECTS OF THE CULTURE

If someone you love has Sante Fe or Tuscan influences in their bedroom this will simply give it a Town and Country touch. It is not Ethnic unless every aspect of the bedroom decoration is Mexican or Italian and probably most of the house is also.

The **female and male Ethnic** bedrooms cannot be described. They depend on the culture represented. There is authenticity when a person reflects the Ethnic style. There is respect for all aspects of the culture.

The **personality of the Ethnic** bedroom owner will come into the other style personality ranges since within the Ethnic style category is the gamut of expression. Some followers of Ethnic will, for example, be Dramatic, some Town and Country, some Romantic etc. If you know the culture, you will be able to interpret the personality. The detail, line, form and colour of the decorative features of the chosen culture will be of paramount importance to them. So expect the fascinated Ethnic to have a loyal and devoted interest in the detail and the nuances of another culture.

Key words: other cultures.

> 'Be exactly who you are. And do it to the maximum.'
> *Isabella Rossellini*

CHAPTER 7

master strokes

...significant simplicities for success

Here are some strategies to enhance your relationship. Have the courage to put in the time and effort. We guarantee you will reap abundant rewards.

Stroke 1. Clear away the clutter

Do you want more love, romance and happier relationships? Be rid of the clutter in your life. How clean, tidy and organised the rooms of your home are, especially your bedroom, speaks volumes about how clean, tidy and organised you are in the rooms of your soul as well as in the corridors of your self-esteem and self-worth.

Stop hanging on. Is there a reason for keeping all those things, or should you have sorted them – and the reasons – out long ago? What about those empty bottles and jars in the kitchen? What about those clothes you know you will never wear again? If you are inclined to keep too many things 'in case they come in handy', you have to be strong with yourself now. We know you want the best for yourself and your partner. That's one of the reasons you are reading this book. It gives you example after example of changes you can make. What a different life you can have. Have you the courage?

Some of you feel comforted by physical clutter. Fine – it can still be well-dusted and rearranged. In your bedroom, keep everything dusted and polished. Clean the skirting boards; dust the light fittings; pull out the chair/drawers etc. and have a spring clean. You will have moved the molecular energy around and that's good. Clean the window. Even move some furniture around. If it doesn't look good in the new position, move it back. It's amazing how your spirits will lift.

A messy and untidy bedroom can belong to any of the styles we have mentioned in Chapter 6, and reflects a person who is disorganised, easygoing about most aspects of their life and a procrastinator. Or perhaps it belongs to the busy person who is trying to do too many things at once, or someone with lots of creative interests and hobbies. Don't put it off. Sort the clutter now – one room at a time. Start with anything on the floor. If it doesn't belong in that room move it to where it does belong, get rid of it or give it away. You don't have to do it all at once but do get started.

How do *you* feel about your bedroom? Is it a general room for dumping everything or a special sanctuary away from everyday worries? Is it a reflection of inner joy, love and harmony, or a room you only use to store clothes and sleep in? Does it reflect how you feel inside or have you never given it a second thought? Do you love going into it just to admire it and relive sensual memories?

EMOTIONAL CLUTTER CAN PERVADE OUR LIVES

Clutter isn't only physical. Emotional clutter can pervade our lives. Until you come to terms with the sorrow, the longings, the resentment, the anger, the hurt from your last love/marriage/

childhood/business dealing, you are swamped by emotional clutter. Forgive yourself, and in time, the other people involved.

Send them love and peace. Until you can do this, you will be bruised and resentful in all areas of you life. By clearing the emotional clutter you will be in charge of your life.

Stroke 2. Begin the creative make-over of your bedroom

It doesn't matter how small your budget or how tiny your bedroom, choose to have it reflect the real you. Sit in it one morning or evening and really look closely at what you have. Notice the colours, the bed linen, the lamps, the bedside tables. Start listing the changes you could make just by changing some colours. If you are frightened of making a ghastly mistake, then choose a neutral background for walls, ceiling and floor and add colour with accessories. Visit homes for sale on 'open for inspection' days for practical examples, or gather magazines to give you new ideas. Make notes when you find a home and bedroom similar to your heart's desire and discuss the situation with your bedroom partner. If he or she is negative about changes suggest very small ones. Don't let their inertia stop you from moving the relationship into sweeter waters.

Change your bedroom around. You probably can't change the position of the bed, but you can change where chests of drawers, a dressing table or a chair are placed. A fresh coat of paint on the walls or furniture will change your bedroom dramatically. Try different sheets on the bed, or perhaps add cushions to your bed. Lots of cushions in harmony with the bedroom and bed linen give the appearance of generosity, a good attribute for the romantic. The colours you choose reveal a lot about how you are feeling. Listen to your intuition on this. Above all, think romance. Think sensuality.

ABOVE ALL, THINK ROMANCE. THINK SENSUALITY

Stand at the door of your bedroom and consider every surface. Perhaps you have a few books on bedside tables or on the chest of drawers. It's a sign of an inquisitive mind. However, a virtual library in the bedroom confuses the purpose of the room.

A mirror is a very good accessory in your bedroom and depending on where you place it and what you do in sight of it, can be very sensual. A mirror anywhere in the room reflects light and energy, enlarges and inspires the imagination. Round mirrors are especially good for enhancing relationships, according to the principles of Feng Shui. Curves are more romantic than straight-edged lines, in Western eyes too. Look at decorating fashions. Mirrored wardrobes are not particularly romantic – these days we enjoy the cocooning effect of smaller bedrooms and don't need a mirrored wall of aluminium doors.

Now you are getting into the creative mode, consider the lighting in your room. Lamps are the most sensual lighting choice. Don't turn on overhead lights or use fluorescent lighting. If you enjoy reading in bed, have good bedside lamps, at the right height. For romance don't always read in bed. If you want to explore the link between colour psychology and lamp choices, realise that a lamp with a pink shade gives the

LAMPS ARE THE MOST SENSUAL LIGHTING CHOICE

colour of love throughout the bedroom; blue creates calm and contentment; green helps with rejuvenation and restoration of energy; mauve and lilac increase the fantasy factor; white or cream lampshades provide soft lighting and harmonise perfectly with the other colours in your room.

Candles certainly create a very sensual mood, but can be dangerous. If you want them in your bedroom, be safe and sensual. Keep them away from curtains and other objects and don't use any candle with a paper cuff around it. It is possible to use candles safely before you get into bed. Have them lit in the bedroom to create the romantic atmosphere you want. Allow the drip to build up. It gives the look of sensuality rather than having a neat and clean candle and candle holder or modern candelabra.

One of the loveliest accessories you can add to your sensual bedroom are fresh flowers. Choose masses of flowers or single beauties to maximise the look of your bedroom retreat. Perhaps you enjoy dried flowers. Go easy on these in your bedroom. They will collect dust from bedcovers and Feng Shui experts maintain they are not conducive to good relationships since they are dead items. We want your relationship to be alive, prosperous and joyous.

> **CHOOSE MASSES OF FLOWERS OR SINGLE BEAUTIES TO MAXIMISE THE LOOK OF YOUR BEDROOM RETREAT**

Whether the look you aim for is cluttered and comfortable, or simple and practical, or elegant, or dramatic, keep your eyes open for accessories to support your desires. First look around your home. Use small items you wouldn't normally associate with bedroom design as decorations. Our friend Bob used his three old leather suitcases stacked on top of each other as storage space for blankets and clothing. He regularly places a single flower tied with a ribbon on the top suitcase. Louise uses brooches and earrings as decorative features on the bedroom wall, attaching them with Blu·Tack and uses one, three or five items grouped together. Odd numbers always give a more interesting look than even numbered items unless you place four to form a square.

Angela, a single friend of ours, uses a hat stand and cane basket to display her sexy underwear, evening gloves and red feather boa, much to the delight of her admirers. The display works on her own sex drive too.

Some people have part of their office in the bedroom. The computer gives a different feel to the room. Where do tasks end and the relationship begin? Get rid of the office (even if it only takes up a small space) if you want romance to blossom. Make your bedroom for sleeping and romancing, not working.

One last thought on bedroom accessories. You decorate your room for yourself and for your partner. So you have a first impression when you walk into the room and a second impression when you sit and lie in bed looking from a different angle. Make sure there is a congruency. What you can see from your bed, what you feel with sheets, pillows and covers underneath you says a lot about you and your attitude to the relationship. Your oasis of love must look and smell clean and fresh whether late at night with lamp light or by early daylight. It's a way to make a fresh start.

Stroke 3. Change the way you do things

Tired of what you've been getting in the romance stakes? Change your modus operandi, not only in the way you communicate with partners and potential partners but more importantly the way you communicate with yourself especially

TIRED OF WHAT YOU'VE BEEN GETTING IN THE ROMANCE STAKES? CHANGE YOUR MODUS OPERANDI

in your bedroom. Once you feel really excited by the appearance of this room of rest and pleasure, your outlook on life and relationships will change too. You really have to want to change.

Carolyn's story

Carolyn, a single woman, changed most aspects of her bedroom while we were writing this book. She wanted a loving and sensual relationship based on mutual respect, warm-heartedness and laughter. Her bedroom became less structured Classic and Town and Country and softer, more pastel, and definitely more Romantic, with Classic and Town and Country overtones.

Instead of straight hanging curtains there are now softly swathed white muslin curtains. Instead of pillow cases with straight edges now there are loose frills on the edges of two out of the four. Carolyn bought and painted new bedside drawers, dismissed the Classic lamp and shade and substituted curved lamp bases with a definite Town and Country texture. She rearranged the pictures in the bedroom, put some in other rooms and introduced a stunning Romantic painting.

Has her love life changed? Yes, because she feels more loving and much happier. She achieved this because she let go of a lot of the clutter in her emotional life.

The changes Carolyn made cost very little. Inexpensive purchases and the recycling of existing accessories made a huge difference and the tiniest dent in her wallet. Carolyn spent time thinking about what to put on the wall, behind and above her as she lay in bed, since she knew this was very important. Why is it?

The decoration on the wall behind your bed symbolises your life as you sleep. It has a subliminal effect on you. It states who you are, what is important to you and your goals in life. What is the significance of the decoration/painting/print hovering above you?

When you choose a plain wall with no embellishments (disregard the bed head) you are uncomplicated, controlled and serious. Nothing unnecessary for you. On the other hand, a mosquito net, whether small or large, hung above the bed, is very romantic. Placing a large mirror on the wall behind the bed (or on the ceiling) is sensual and erotic and certainly an invitation to look at yourself.

Moving completely away from the self-fascinated is the person who places the bed under a window with uninterrupted views to the outside.

> **A MOSQUITO NET, WHETHER SMALL OR LARGE, HUNG ABOVE THE BED, IS VERY ROMANTIC**

What an adventure-loving, outgoing, down-to-earth person. A practical person may place the bed under a window with only a view of the wall next door. After all, the bed is for sleeping and sex. Life is reality and if your bedroom doesn't have a wonderful view, it's nothing to get upset about.

Perhaps you have a painting of a beautiful nude or something erotic and sexually stimulating on that wall behind your head? Sensuality and sexuality are obviously abiding passions for you awake and asleep. Many people hang a favourite painting on the wall behind the bed. A happy picture of flowers suggests an optimistic outlook. A scene talks to you about dreams and desires. What are your dreams and desires?

What did Carolyn place on her wall? She wanted a loving relationship, so she decided on a garland of cream and peach coloured roses with green leaves as the background. The garland came to life with the addition of a light golden bow with long ribbons. It is reminiscent of a marriage garland. So now last thing at night, Carolyn can look up at the flowers and salute the love in her life, the intertwining of symbols and the beauty above her.

Stroke 4. Remedies for the bedroom

The bedroom can be a place of rejuvenation, relaxation, nurturing, comfort, security, safety and love as well as sensual and sexual gratification.

- If you are looking for contentment and security, decorate with blues.
- If it is rejuvenation and relaxation you most need in your bedroom, use green.
- If physical love is your need, choose pink.
- If you wish to improve the communication between your partner and yourself, choose peach or apricot.
- For an underactive sex life, add some red to the room – be subtle, don't overdo it or you won't be able to sleep afterwards!
- If an overactive sex life is leaving you exhausted, add some green to the room to create more balance. This could be in the form of pot plants if you don't want to add green in other ways.

You don't need to paint the walls in these colours, although some of you may choose to. All you have to do is add touches of the colours listed above. Perhaps your new sheets, pillowcases and bedcover will reflect these changes. The more 'touches', the more your commitment to the desired outcome.

When you share a bedroom with a partner, whose style predominates? Does it matter to you? Perhaps it's an indication of who has the most control in the relationship and especially in terms of the sexual component. Many men let their partner be the decorator and designer. They feel women have a better eye for colour and style detail. This is not always true, so you should listen to your mate. With this book in your hand, discuss what you both want intimately and how best it can be achieved.

IF YOU UNDERSTAND THE PSYCHOLOGICAL MESSAGES OF YOUR CHOICE OF COLOUR AND STYLE, YOU CAN DISCUSS WHERE YOU WOULD LIKE TO BE IN YOUR RELATIONSHIP

Compromise is the best way to decide on bedroom decor. If you understand the psychological messages of your choice of colour and style, you can discuss where you would like to be in your relationship and choose the options with this in mind. If you like different colours, perhaps one colour can be used as the main colour and the other as an accent.

The ensuite bathroom

If you have an ensuite bathroom adjacent to the bedroom, it's part of your relationship too. It is an extension of your bedroom, only used by the two of you, leads off your private sensual domain and so is part of your intimate and private life. Water relates strongly to emotions. The bathroom can be a place of great cleansing, emotionally and physically. It is not uncommon for both men and women to retreat to the bathroom for privacy and tears.

So make the ensuite as welcoming and comfortable as possible, make the presence of water a charming seducer. Keep the bathroom spotlessly clean because clean is inviting. Give some thought to the colours of towels and accessories. This is a relationship area. What do you want your relationship to represent?

Do you have a sterile no decoration, ensuite bathroom? That says a lot about the uncomplicated life you want. Life is never as uncomplicated as that. Putting in some shells or plants may well change your relationship and allow you to see things differently.

Think softness if you desire more romance and intimacy. Perhaps something draped will achieve it. Perhaps the colours of towels will do it. Look once more at Chapter 5 for colour meanings and ideas. Pastels are softening, deep colours with contrast are more dramatic and medium colours suggest just that, a medium and confident look at life.

THINK SOFTNESS IF YOU DESIRE MORE ROMANCE AND INTIMACY.

If you rent or can't afford changes just yet, you can still use some colour in a variety of ways – move a plant from another area of the house, buy a new shower curtain, collect a few shells and display them, and most of all clear away the clutter. Yes here we go again. Get rid of the clutter from your life by cleaning the shelves and drawers of the bathroom cupboards, and we guarantee you will improve your outlook on life.

Stroke 5. What to wear to bed

Now we are getting really personal. Some of you have already answered, *nothing*. So perhaps we can rephrase the question. What do you wear as or before you get into bed?
- What is the style of your nightwear?
- What colours do you feel best in?

Let's take a look at the popular meanings behind your choice as you prepare for bed.

Women

- Do you prefer to wear short and sexy pyjamas? You probably need to feel secure in your relationship, as you did as a child. You want a partner who is strong and protective.
- Are you the sexy, mysterious black lace type? You are in control and ready to seduce your man into a web of love and sensuality by wearing black suspender belt and black stockings before bed. At other times the black nightgown will more than suffice. Not only are you seductive and sexual, you also love to be seduced in a dramatic way.

> **ARE YOU THE SEXY, MYSTERIOUS BLACK LACE TYPE?**

- Are you the fashion-conscious type who must wear designer or trendy clothes? It will be the same with nightwear for you — only the best and the latest styles will do. You are ambitious, strong-willed and determined, with a lot of energy. This is reflected in your intimate life as well.

> **NOT ONLY ARE YOU SEDUCTIVE AND SEXUAL, YOU ALSO LOVE TO BE SEDUCED IN A DRAMATIC WAY**

- If long silk or satin nightgowns in white or pastels, with perhaps lace added, are your favourite, you are a tactile, sensitive person who loves to be appreciated. You enjoy thoughtful and romantic foreplay.
- You adore your pretty, floral, somewhat sheer nightgown. It tells your partner you want a loving, sensual relationship, including tender caresses and lots of cuddling.
- Love the comfy pyjamas or nightshirt? You are so practical and down-to-earth, and security is important. You are not very spontaneous although there is a sexual plan to follow when you choose.
- If you prefer to wear a T-shirt, you are a sporty and practical person who likes freedom of movement in clothing. You are

PERHAPS YOU PREFER TO WEAR HIS PYJAMAS! YOU REALLY WANT INTIMACY DON'T YOU? usually fairly confident sexually. You know what you want!

- Perhaps you prefer to wear his pyjamas! You really want intimacy don't you? This move is fine for a surprise, just don't do it too often. You will be giving away your own personality too much.
- You prefer to wear nothing. You have a confident and strong personality, are competitive and positive in life and in your relationships. Adventure and spontaneity are important to you, and you like wandering around the house naked.
- Those who deliberately dab on their favourite perfume and wear nothing but perfume before bed are strong and confident and feminine. Romance is important to you.

Our research indicates most men prefer a woman to wear sexy nightwear to bed rather than nothing at all. They prefer to have something left to their imagination. It increases arousal. Once in bed, undressing each other is part of the sensual pleasure.

MOST MEN PREFER A WOMAN TO WEAR SEXY NIGHT WEAR TO BED RATHER THAN NOTHING AT ALL

Choose colours for nightwear to enhance your own colouring. The most seductive and sensual colours for women to wear to bed are:

- black – mysterious and seductive
- red – very sexual
- pink – gentle, loving and sensual (for those with cool colour skin undertones)
- peach – gentle, communicative and sensual (good for those with warm colour skin undertones)
- white – pure and chaste

Research has found that men respond favourably to peach and apricot colours in particular on women, and they love red!

Men

What do you wear before you get into bed?
- Men who wear pyjamas (tops and bottoms) tend to be conventional, practical and down-to-earth. They are not the spontaneous type but certainly know what they like.
- If you wear just the pyjama bottoms (whether long or short legged) you are more physical and sensual but still very practical.
- Silk or silk-like boxer shorts are very different. These are chosen for a reason. You are tactile and sensual, loving the feel of the silkiness against your skin. You are quite a romantic and certainly aware of fashion.
- The underpants and T-shirt wearer is very practical. You feel comfortable with these, can toss the covers off, get up in the night, even answer the door and at all times feel in control.
- If you wear underpants only, you are heading towards freedom, or perhaps you have children around and you would really prefer no clothes but that's not realistic. You feel you need at all times to protect your most precious asset.
- Nothing. Men who prefer to wear nothing but their birthday suits as they prepare for bed are confident, competitive and very sexual.

What colours do women respond to when a man is preparing for bed? Not pastels, nor the ever favourite light blue pyjamas which are good for sleeping, but not for seduction. Choose instead stronger colours such as

CHOOSE STRONGER COLOURS SUCH AS BURGUNDY, RED, BLACK, NAVY OR DEEP GREEN

burgundy, red, black, navy or deep green (not brown, no turn-on there). Even medium colours will have more sexual interest than the pastels. Experiment. Find out for yourself.

Do you wear socks to bed? Or a head covering? Or a track suit?

Obviously, these items of warm clothing are not romantic. They make getting sensual with you difficult. If you want your life to change in the near future, change your attitude to your body. Don't feel defensive because we have identified your 'security blanket'. If you want a more romantic life, discard these items and substitute a different method of keeping yourself warm. Experiment, whether you are on your own or not. Turn up the electric blanket for a little longer if you need to. Of course there are some winter nights when you need as much covering as possible.

If you suffer from cold feet by all means wear socks to sleep in, but not for sex! If you suffer from cramps and cold feet, put a hot water bottle in the bed to warm your toes and involve your mate with it too. Or have a warm bath or shower before bed. Not every night is for romance and sex but having a loving and approachable body next to yours does wonders for companionship.

Stroke 6. Romancing and seducing each style

How can you improve the romance and sex in your relationship? By understanding how each style likes to be wooed. Have another look at Chapter 6, then enjoy some very enlightening advice from the following ideas.

Master Strokes

Men and women interpret sexual moves and seduction techniques differently. What is normal behaviour for some could be seen by others as confronting and compromising. The tactics you choose to seduce are probably very different from those used by your friends and acquaintances. Interestingly, we never talk about these step-by-step intimate details even to our closest friends because they are our own private techniques and with each partner they vary slightly. These are the processes we have found work for us over the years: the body language, the pauses, the lingering, the smiles, the flirting, the haste and the words which are our fingerprints of technique.

The good news is you can keep doing those flirtatious behaviours, but now you can add something else which will give you unparalleled success. We have knowledge for you to make the path from A to Z intriguingly seductive. When you begin to demonstrate how much pleasure you can give, you will find your partner responding too. These strategies work equally well for a new romance as for a long-term romance. Put away the bitterness, the anger, the hurt and the regrets if you want more romance in your life. Lift your relationship out of its predictable and boring state. Here are some ideas to assist you to become a splendid seducer.

The first task is to identify the personality style of your partner, remembering that combinations of two styles are the most common. Think about what your partner wears and how he or she decorates the home. The more you understand your partner, the greater the chance for success. Romance is not just sex. It is a relationship. So notice how your partner lives. The way the

> **THE MORE YOU UNDERSTAND YOUR PARTNER, THE GREATER THE CHANCE FOR SUCCESS**

home is arranged, kept clean and tidy, the internal and external appearance of the car (not the choice and model) speaks volumes about confidence, self-esteem and most importantly for us, their preferred bedroom style in decoration and ultimately in behaviour. Become familiar with the nine styles described in Chapter 6.

When we discuss combinations of styles we mean two *major* styles. Some people are very definitely one style, but most are two. When you look closely at a bedroom and a house you can often see aspects of each of the nine styles represented. Which style or styles predominate?

This is relatively simple if you are in the early stages of a romance. Take a peek at the bedroom. If you live together and you both had some say in the decoration of the bedroom, scrutinise carefully your partner's input. Identify the style or styles they prefer in this most intimate of rooms. Often the accessories used will give you the guide you need.

SUCCESS COMES FROM THE SIMPLEST IDEAS Use the romantic strategies described below to seduce your partner. Success comes from the simplest ideas. Mastery is the key.

CLASSIC

The Classic personality is conventional, controlled, but does like a touch of the dramatic to excite them. She or he likes to be treated with style. An elegant and classy restaurant is preferred – everything about a good restaurant, such as the way the menu is designed, the quality background music, the decoration of the table, the behaviour of the waiters and waitresses, fits with the Classic's idea of charming behaviour. Deference and consideration are very important. No noisy arguments, no clatter from the kitchen, life should be sweet and charming.

The Classic person prefers to know what the ritual is going to be. They don't particularly enjoy surprises because they like everything in its right place, including sex. Sex is to be savoured, not rushed. Classic women and men are detail conscious. They love to be appreciated and adored for themselves, their organisational skills and their well functioning life. Control of all things keeps them happy. They don't aim to control their partner, merely to understand what is going to happen next, so in their mind everything is neat and tidy.

Meaningless sex is difficult for them. Being reserved, loving and affectionate, they respond to tenderness and sincerity in their loving relationships. Respect is an important aspect of their sex life.

What can you do to seduce the **Classic woman**? Take her to that stylish restaurant. Entertain her with style, wearing colour coordinated, appropriate tailored clothing. Bring her flowers. Tell her how elegant she always looks. Have soft music in the background. Ensure your bedroom is neat and tidy and smells fresh. Good champagne with lovely glasses to take to the bedroom, interesting sex using more than the missionary position in bed, and an unusual breakfast the next morning will impress her.

Don't expect her to get her fingernails dirty. Camping is not a good getaway for this woman who wants to have a hair dryer handy as well as her make-up, and a bed which can be straightened each day.

And remember not to look messy in bed the next morning. She won't. She will creep out of bed to do her hair, clean her teeth, perhaps even put on very light and natural make-up. Keep up to her standards. This is a feminine woman, in fact sometimes quite demure and modest.

When your purpose is to seduce the **Classic man**, remember he is elegant, sophisticated and poised. He likes a little drama and excitement in his sex life, but done tastefully. Begin the seduction process by taking him to a lovely restaurant, or with a formal dinner for two at home, even complete with silver candelabra and classical music. Love and commitment are important to the organised male. Be sure to take care of the little things when planning a seduction. Make sure there are no loose ends, because if you don't see them, he will.

> **LOVE AND COMMITMENT ARE IMPORTANT TO THE ORGANISED MALE**

Good news: still waters run deep.

DRAMATIC

The Dramatic's bedroom style, with its use of colour and theatrical accessories tells you a lot about their sensual and sexual style. To satisfy the Dramatic man or woman's whims in seduction, include some extreme and dramatic settings or behaviours.

There is nothing ordinary or conventional about the **Dramatic woman**. Do not treat her like a Classic. She will be thoroughly bored. That sort of behaviour is too conventional for her. She may like to shock you and to be shocked by you as well, so to seduce her, explicit sexual

> **THERE IS NOTHING ORDINARY OR CONVENTIONAL ABOUT THE DRAMATIC WOMAN**

talk is a turn-on, along with unusual behaviour. The unpredictable is also exciting for her, with no rules or regulations. Suggest going for a ride on a motorbike, having a meal of oysters and French bread washed down with something cool, then retiring to bed with black leathers to be unzipped slowly.

Passion and excitement are the way she likes relationships to be. Take her to elegant or stylishly modern restaurants, dress up for the occasion in striking clothes and excite her imagination by suggesting unusual lovemaking positions.

The **Dramatic male** loves an exciting and adventurous sex life without rules and regulations. He enjoys lust and sensuality, sometimes to the point of being animalistic. That explains why both male and female Dramatics often have fabrics with animal prints in the bedroom. To the Dramatic male, sex is a pleasure to be savoured. It is an adventure. Be unpredictable and he will love it. Have the black or red suspenders and stocking ritual down to a fine art, with a rose between the teeth and a feather boa for added drama. Passion is a necessary stimulant to his sex life. When you are aiming to seduce him, take him to an exotic restaurant or cook him colourful and creative dishes. Decorate your table with strong or bright colours. Keep it simple and angled as opposed to curved with flower arrangements.

BE UNPREDICTABLE AND HE WILL LOVE IT

Good news: drama is 'sexciting'.

ROMANTIC

The Romantic person's bedroom has lots of curves in decoration, and in design for bed linen. So your strategy is sensuality. Romantics think and breathe sensuality all the time:

in their touching behaviours towards you, in the way they dress and undress, in the way they make the bed and in their attitude to setting the table and cooking food. The **Romantic woman** loves the full romantic seduction ritual and she is ready for it most days. Start in the morning with loving suggestions and perhaps a phone call during the day if you are at work. Make sensual and enticing suggestions of what may happen later in the day. Dinner at a romantic restaurant, with dimmed lights and a seductive atmosphere, or perhaps a lovely view of city lights or moonlight over water is enough to set her pulse racing. Remember the flowers and there is nothing like red or pink roses to set the scene. If dining at home, choose romantic music, definitely dim the lights and create a sensual bedroom with perhaps rose petals scattered in the bed. Take your time, don't rush the foreplay. Long and sensual is an important part of the ritual. Soft, tender caresses increase the passion. Undress her slowly and admire out loud what you see.

> IF DINING AT HOME, CHOOSE ROMANTIC MUSIC, DEFINITELY DIM THE LIGHTS AND CREATE A SENSUAL BEDROOM WITH PERHAPS ROSE PETALS SCATTERED IN THE BED

The **Romantic man** also enjoys being treated in a very sensual way. Take a lot of care in planning dinners and special events. Cook dinner for him and invite him to taste as you cook, to be close to you in the kitchen. Get him involved so he can be touched and kissed as the cooking is bubbling along. If you dine out, choose an elegant and romantic restaurant, with good atmosphere and subdued lighting or candles. Foreplay is very important. He enjoys the slow seduction process enormously. Expect your underwear to tell him a lot about your intentions.

Make it revealing, have a sense of delicacy and choose pastels or white. You will be good at being coy. Wear alluring perfume, tease him a little and breathe heavily when you are near. And in bed, take your time. Whisper sweet words in his ear and plan how sensual you can be.

Good news: romance is around every curve.

Town and Country

The Town and Country style is more casual and comfortable than the others we have discussed so far. Relaxing country style is preferred. The log fire, home style cooking, baking, flowers in unusual vases (perhaps an old jug), lots of soft pillows are all high on the list for Town and Country people. A weekend in the country is another option. Touching is an important part of the seduction process for the Town and Country personality. They are very tactile. They tend to be rather cautious until they feel secure with their partner, and then they become dedicated and committed lovers.

> **Touching is an important part of the seduction process for the Town and Country personality**

When you want to seduce a **Town and Country woman**, have the smells of delicious cooking in the kitchen, the feel and smell of clean linen in the bathroom and bedroom, use flower essences such as lavender and gardenia around the home in pot pourri, have the constant appearance of homeliness and comfortable lounges to cuddle up on.

Take this forthright natural woman to a comfortable restaurant with tables lit by candles. Be sure there is comfort food on the menu such as soups, crusty bread, honest meat and vegetable dishes and lots of salads and vegetable combinations. Be certain too that the dessert menu includes such fancies as sticky date pudding, egg custards, bread and butter puddings, berry crumbles, apple pies and fruit platters.

Speak honestly and openly about your emotions. She will love to comfort you by touching. She is a good friend, even if the relationship is going nowhere. You can depend on her.

The Town and Country man is very tactile, so touch him a lot. Once secure in the relationship he becomes a dedicated and committed lover. Take him to a more casual restaurant, with a log fire and a country atmosphere, or better still, start the seduction process early in the day and take him for a drive into the country to a genuine country restaurant. He'll love it.

Good news: do you want a massage?

CONTEMPORARY

The Contemporary style is based on simplicity, clean lines and vibrant colours. Shiny smooth surfaces, minimal decoration, angular rather than curved shapes, with unusual combinations of bright colours, is typical of their style. Similar to the Dramatics, but much more relaxed, these people are not detail conscious, preferring a minimalist decor, free of clutter and extraneous objects.

The Contemporary style can initially appear aloof, but they really love to be with people. They are very sensitive, caring and friendly when you get to know them. In interpersonal relationships they prefer the direct approach, so say what you mean. They love to be seduced and romanced, but not fussed over. They love spontaneity and surprises, so don't seduce

THEY LOVE SPONTANEITY AND SURPRISES

in the same way each time as they'll get bored with it. Flexibility and freedom in their sex lives is important. This doesn't mean flexibility and freedom with different partners, as they tend to be very loyal in a long-term relationship.

Above all, Contemporaries love to have fun. Make them laugh, joke about sex, seduce them with pleasure. They love the playful approach. When they bring the stresses of the day home, as they often do, listen to them, empathise, then gently lighten them up and make them laugh. Go to a restaurant that is simple, modern and classy in decor. It must be trendy with simple and elegant, yet tasty, food. Roughing it is not the best way to seduce a Contemporary.

Seduction should begin in a fun way, either early in the day with a humorous invitation or with some sexual bantering and innuendo. In the bedroom, fresh, clean sheets, perhaps satin, are essential. Create a sensual atmosphere with the use of soft lighting. Continue the sexual banter to set the mood.

The **female Contemporary** enjoys a gift of unusual flowers such as orchids, lilies, tulips or bird of paradise to precede the seduction process. Whisper suggestive comments in her ear during the day or leave suggestive notes in places where she will find them. Keep it simple and unusual. Surprise her. Foreplay is important but it should not be an elaborate and detailed process. Find out what she likes and do it!

> **WHISPER SUGGESTIVE COMMENTS IN HER EAR DURING THE DAY OR LEAVE SUGGESTIVE NOTES IN PLACES WHERE SHE WILL FIND THEM**

The **Contemporary male** creates a simple and uncomplicated lifestyle at home to allow himself more time out with others. He loves lots of fun and pleasure in his leisure time. Take him to an amusement park or a comedy movie or somewhere he can let his hair down and laugh. That will put him in the best mood for the rest of the evening and the pleasures you have in store for him. Keep seduction light-hearted for this man.

Good news: spontaneity and light-heartedness brings happy rewards.

Practical

Simple styling, with no extremes in decoration and nothing too elaborate, reflects the Practical person. These people are down-to-earth, natural and uncomplicated. The casual, functional, no-frills look is theirs. It is a look which is balanced, neat and tidy, and comfortable. They are a very casual version of the Classic style, with some Town and Country influence as well. Practicals are caring and considerate but often methodical and analytical in their ways, rather than spontaneous. They like the predictable, they like to know what is going to happen and when.

The seduction process should be kept simple and natural, not contrived or forced. They enjoy sex when it happens, but it doesn't have a high priority as practical issues always take precedence. Practicals can easily fall into habitual patterns in their sex life and can become predictable and boring in a long-term relationship. They might like to have sex on the same day, at the same time and in the same way each week. If this is the case, find out if there is another style that is also part of

> **PRACTICALS CAN EASILY FALL INTO HABITUAL PATTERNS IN THEIR SEX LIFE AND CAN BECOME PREDICTABLE AND BORING IN A LONG-TERM RELATIONSHIP**

their personality and use elements of that style to boost your sex life. Keep foreplay simple and relaxed, and don't rush it.

For a night out, a simple restaurant is all that is needed. They like classy but unpretentious eateries. Practicals are mindful of the cost of the night out. They are the bargain hunters of the world and like value for money, so extravagance can often embarrass them. Home style cooking with traditional country style comfort food is inviting to them. Always have a dessert. They love it and no meal is complete to them without it. Keep the dinner table simple and neat, with only the necessary items on the table.

For the **female Practical**, the best way to a successful evening of seduction begins earlier in the day when you help with the housework. Help her with the dishes or the cooking, vacuum for her, assist her with the practical duties she must complete before she can relax and receive pleasure. With your help, she will not be so tired at the end of the day and more willing to participate in a sexual adventure. A potted flowering plant rather than fresh flowers is a good way to show her you care. Her practical nature may think flowers a waste of money. An appropriate gift of her favourite chocolates from time to time will also be well received. Don't expect her to wear romantic lacy underwear and lingerie. It will be simple, comfortable, practical and clean, in basic colours of neutrals such as white, beige or grey, or in blues or greens. Turn down the lights to create a soft subtle atmosphere. Be loving to her, get her in the mood for pleasure. Perhaps a gentle massage, to remove the stresses of her day. Keep foreplay simple, but don't rush it. Once she is relaxed, she will enjoy whatever you have in mind for her.

Responsibilities weigh heavy for the **Practical man**. Lighten his load if you can. Of course he enjoys sex (what man doesn't) but can become set in his ways. Get him out of his pyjamas and break his normal going to bed routine. Comfort and security are the basis of his existence. Sometimes stir the pot. The Practical man might not know how to get out of the usual routine, so you'll have to be the one to vary it. Use your imagination and creative abilities to inspire changes in foreplay and seduction with him. Show him there are other ways – he will enjoy it. Begin his seduction by encouraging him to stop working a little earlier than normal for one day. The world won't fall apart just this once. Prepare his favourite meal at home and remember his favourite dessert. That's sure to put him in the right mood. Spontaneity is uncomfortable for him, so preparation is the key to success. Tell him what you have planned so he can get used to the idea first. Make it special, but not too far out of his comfort zone.

> **USE YOUR IMAGINATION AND CREATIVE ABILITIES TO INSPIRE CHANGES IN FOREPLAY AND SEDUCTION WITH HIM**

Good news: share the tasks, plan the seduction and you are in for a good time.

CREATIVE

Flair, style, unusual colour combinations and creative fabric are the elements which set the Creatives apart from the rest. These are the non-conformists among us. They tend to mix a little of everything to create their own individual style. Fabrics with patterns, fabrics with fringes and tassels, scarves and sarongs are basic decorating items to a Creative. Often they will decorate their homes with their own quirky and unusual art pieces, and they may even screen print their own fabrics to use in their homes and clothing. Admire their artwork, and ask them to explain it to you. They will love it.

Unusual restaurants are the norm for them, nothing classic and ordinary. Cult restaurants with eclectic colourful decor may well appeal. Unusual food combinations presented in a casual, relaxed style will seduce them. This doesn't mean they don't like traditional family cooking, they just like to experience different cuisine when they go out. If entertaining at home they may decorate the table with a mixture of odd cutlery, crockery and serviettes with many different shapes and colours. Table centrepieces may be created by combining unrelated items from their stock of odd collectibles. Unusual candles will nearly always be a feature. The food they serve may be non-traditional, or it may be traditional style with combinations you would not normally think to put together.

With seduction, think unique, different, unusual, new. Combine different elements. Be spontaneous. The more variety the better. Surprise them with your ingenuity. Creatives don't like habitual rituals. In the bedroom, ensure the bed looks comfortable and inviting. Ruffle the cover a little, throw a piece of fabric or a scarf over the lamps to mute the light and send colour throughout the room. Or use coloured light globes to throw a sensual glow throughout the room. Be aware of the different and unusual atmosphere you are creating.

> **WITH SEDUCTION, THINK UNIQUE, DIFFERENT, UNUSUAL, NEW. COMBINE DIFFERENT ELEMENTS**

The **female Creative** is the free spirit who often shocks the traditional Classics and Practicals. Be innovative when seducing her. Think of feathers and other titillating tools. Change your seduction style each time and vary the body positions. Surprise her, don't bore her.

The **Creative man** loves spontaneity. Send him intriguing notes, seduce him with the unusual. Variety is the spice of life for him. As long as you do it with a sense of flair, anything goes. Don't be shy with him. Drape yourself in seductive fabric. Let his imagination whirl.

Good news: unique, quirky, has colourful flair.

FANTASY

This personality is the dreamer and the idealist. They are the escapists of this world. Their fantasy is based on either the past or the future. It may embrace the ethereal world of fairies, the celebrity world of Hollywood or the celestial realms of the cosmos. If you are in a relationship with a Fantasy style, talk to them about their fantasy, find out what it is that appeals to them. Whatever you do, don't ridicule them if you don't understand them. Allow them their dreams. They are often quite creative people who just prefer not to relate to the mundane world.

THE ROAD TO SEDUCTION FOR THIS PERSONALITY IS ONE BUILT ON THE IMAGINATION

The road to seduction for this personality is one built on the imagination. Paint exotic mind pictures related to their type of fantasy style. Include their fantasy style in the seduction. They love to experiment during sex, to soar to great heights, although sometimes those heights are unrealistic. They like to remove themselves from day-to-day life. Go along for the ride.

Go to a restaurant that has elements like their fantasy if you can find one. If her bedroom is based on fairies, choose a soft romantic restaurant, with reminiscences of the past. If it has a *Star Wars* theme, choose a restaurant that has shiny surfaces, with red, grey, black or chrome and stainless steel. If it is heavenly, with lots of moons and stars, choose a restaurant with large windows through which you can see the stars in the night sky. A fantasy based on Hollywood movie icons gives you the option of going to any restaurant whose walls are lined with memorabilia of old movie themes and stars.

Sex for the **female Fantasy** style can be a gentle sensual experience, or an exotic adventure. They need a partner who is sensitive, caring, playful, trustworthy and free of limitations. The sense of universal connection with everything in their life is often what motivates them.

The **male Fantasy** personality is usually interested in the future. Of course, Elvis Presley, the rocking rolling 1950s or the Art Deco era may have some followers as well. Sex for these men is always an adventure. Be innovative, straight-forward and introduce elements of their fantasy into the seduction.

Good news: the fantasy adds interesting spice.

ETHNIC

The Ethnic personality is based on one or more of the other styles, with decoration of the bedroom totally based on a particular culture. It could reflect a passion for Mexico, Bali, Japan, Italy, Greece, Spain or any other country. Whatever the interest, there will be objects and artefacts from that culture evident in the decorative aspects of the bedroom. Someone choosing to use a style from

THEY DREAM OF FARAWAY PLACES. THEY LOVE TO TRAVEL

a culture other than their own is usually romantic and into some fantasy. They dream of faraway places. They love to travel. They differ from those who choose their own ethnic cultural style when residing in another country.

Ethnic style personalities live and breathe the culture they love, so take them to a restaurant which is very authentic in its style, or prepare a romantic dinner at home with elements of decoration from their preferred culture as well as an authentic menu.

> **LEARN SOME LOVING AND ROMANTIC WORDS AND PHRASES FROM THAT CULTURE AND SURPRISE THEM WHEN THEY LEAST EXPECT IT BY WRITING A LOVE NOTE OR OFFERING AN INVITATION IN THAT LANGUAGE**

Find out about the intricacies of their favourite culture and base your seduction on acceptable standards in that culture. Learn some loving and romantic words and phrases from that culture and surprise them when they least expect it by writing a love note or offering an invitation in that language. Whatever you do, you will win them over by being authentic in your approach.

As the Ethnic personality will also be one of the other styles already discussed, it will be up to you to decide the combination. For example, a lover of Spanish decor will most likely be a Dramatic–Romantic combination. Follow the seduction ideas for both those styles. If your partner loves the Italian Tuscan look, then Town and Country will be the basic style. If Japanese is their passion, Dramatic or Contemporary will be the seduction style to follow.

Good news: enjoy the journey to faraway places.

Afterplay

After the seduction and sex, consider the power of continuing the romance for a few minutes more while in that wonderful state of love. Afterplay is almost as important as foreplay. It doesn't last as long, but it is just as necessary and satisfying. If you roll over and go to sleep immediately, the afterglow diminishes.

AFTERPLAY IS ALMOST AS IMPORTANT AS FOREPLAY

You have lots of choices for comforting after play. Try some of these to complete the seduction process:
- cuddling
- talking, stroking and touching
- falling asleep comfortably in one another's arms
- enjoying a glass a wine
- perhaps you can think of another.

**Success comes from the simplest ideas.
Mastery is the key.**

SECTION four

living the Sensual and romantic life

'How do I love thee? Let me count the ways.'

Elizabeth Barrett Browning

CHAPTER 8

the golden rules

... creating loving, intimate relationships

By following the suggestions we have made in this book you can make a difference in your intimate relationships. It is all up to you. You are in charge of your life. It's time for new beginnings. Put aside the excuses. Let bygones be bygones and don't let past hurts destroy the present for you. There is a wonderfully colourful future ahead.

> YESTERDAY IS A MEMORY,
> TOMORROW IS A PROMISE,
> TODAY IS A GIFT,
> THAT'S WHY IT'S CALLED ... THE PRESENT
> (Anonymous)

Make a date with yourself to create the happiest and most loving life you can. Set the actual day and put it in your diary. Promise yourself from that day on you *will* be more sensual, more romantic, more thoughtful and more loving. Don't wait, do it now while all the information in this book is fresh in your mind.

APART FROM BASIC SURVIVAL NEEDS, LOVE IS THE MOST IMPORTANT ELEMENT IN LIFE

Apart from basic survival needs, love is the most important element in life. Don't waste a minute more without it. Use this book to make positive changes in your intimate life. Have fun with it. Put laughter into your personal relationships.

Living, loving, learning and laughing is what a successful life is about. Make sure you incorporate all four into your life experiences each day. There is a universal plan for all of us and we will be directed to it if we take the time to listen to our inner voice.

The Nine Golden Rules for creating loving intimate relationships

RULE 1: KNOW YOURSELF

A good base to work from is to get in touch with the real and authentic you. Who are you? Activate your senses by discovering what colours you love, what sounds excite you, what scents inspire you, what foods you really love, what textures soothe you. Think about the places you love to go, the types of movies and books you enjoy, the music that makes you laugh and the music that brings tears to your eyes, and the lands you'd love to travel to. What would you like your life to be like in three, five and ten years time? Spend a day alone with yourself. You are important. Know yourself inside out, backwards and forwards, and in every way. Re-read

ACCEPT ALL YOUR POSITIVE ATTRIBUTES AND BE PREPARED TO WORK ON ELIMINATING THE NEGATIVES

Chapter 6 to refresh your ideas on your intimate style. Accept all your positive attributes and be prepared to work on eliminating the negatives. Then move forward into creating the best life for yourself you can.

RULE 2: KNOW YOUR PARTNER

Accept your partner as he or she is. You can't change anyone but yourself, so don't try. We all have agendas that others can't relate to. This is normal and part of being human.

Learn everything you can about your partner. Understand his or her intimate style and the seduction techniques you can use. Discover what stimulates his or her senses when it comes to colours, sounds, scents, foods and textures. Develop a list of your partner's favourite flowers, chocolates, cars, sports, songs, singers, movies, foods, fruits, vegetables, desserts and so on, so you can use the information for romantic, loving interludes. Know your loved one's clothing sizes, including underwear and lingerie sizes.

Rule 3: Commitment

You *both* have to be committed to a loving long-lasting relationship or there is no hope of success. Discuss it. Ensure you both want the same thing. Commitment means putting your relationship ahead of everything else in your life, at the top of your priority list. It means being faithful to the partnership, supportive of your partner and enthusiastic about the relationship. It means working through the pain that inevitably occurs in any relationship, to find the pot of gold at the end.

Rule 4: Be honest about the state of your relationship

Is it really good as it is? If your answer is 'yes', congratulations. Keep doing more of what you're doing and perhaps take some ideas from this book to keep the partnership fresh.

If your answer is 'no', are you at the boredom stage? Then it's time to shake up the partnership and revamp it. Read Chapter 2,

'The Seducer's Notebook' and begin romancing all over again. If your sex life is in the doldrums, reread all three chapters in Section 3 to bring new energy to your bedroom and to your sensual and intimate life.

Rule 5. Communication

Listen, talk, share, communicate. Don't run away from your problems nor bury your head in the sand. Nagging by a female partner is a warning sign of problems. Avoiding time at home and with you is a warning sign from a male partner. Find out what the problem is. Don't assume you know what your partner is thinking. Ask. Negotiate. Talk about what irritates you, without becoming over-critical, and without becoming defensive. This is the time to be honest in every way. Communicate, clear up misunderstandings, and don't let the sun go down without making up after a disagreement. The silent treatment serves no purpose in a committed relationship.

DON'T ASSUME YOU KNOW WHAT YOUR PARTNER IS THINKING

Rule 6: Compromise

This is important in any relationship. You can't both have everything your own way all the time and be in a loving and sharing relationship. Just make sure one person doesn't give in to the other every time. Take it in turns, or go with the one to whom the choice is most important on that occasion.

Rule 7: Develop shared recreational activities and common goals

Finding common interests is imperative for maintaining a long-lasting, loving relationship. This is the one quality that most long-term marriages have in common. If you have no leisure activities you share at the moment, talk about it, find at least one. It may be bushwalking, gardening, ballroom dancing, investing in the share market together, doing a course together at the local community centre or joining the local art society.

FINDING COMMON INTERESTS IS IMPERATIVE FOR MAINTAINING A LONG-LASTING, LOVING RELATIONSHIP

Sharing common purposes and goals keeps a relationship close too. You may have the common goal of fixing the back garden, so you both need to plan and work on that; or buying a new car, so you both decide what has to happen to achieve it; or moving house; or buying a new refrigerator; or going on a family holiday; or painting the kitchen. Keep common objectives to the fore by placing your steps of progress and ultimate goal on your refrigerator. Talk about the steps and when you achieve the goal, celebrate. This is most important. Then choose your next goal. The more of these activities you share, the more you will have to talk about when you are together and the more you will enjoy one another's company.

RULE 8: TREAT YOUR RELATIONSHIP AS SPECIAL

Don't take your partner for granted. Show love in as many different ways as possible. Not sickly-sweet love, but caring and thoughtful love. Spend time together, find new interests to share, communicate on a deeper level, share your feelings and your dreams, become best friends. Be **SHOW LOVE IN AS MANY DIFFERENT WAYS AS POSSIBLE** enthusiastic. Bring laughter back into every day. Take pride in your appearance, for yourself and your partner. Be the best 'you' possible. Aim to make a difference in your partner's life. Make a renewed commitment to one another or re-affirm your wedding vows. Increase your sensuality and romance your partner all over again and again and again.

Rule 9: Earn Respect, Admiration and Love

Relationships are often hard work, but they are the basis of a happy and worthwhile life. Respect, admiration and love are all earned. Trust and honesty are essential fundamentals. These qualities don't come automatically. You have to prove you deserve them. Show your love, without expecting anything in return. Give affection freely and often. Take a risk in disclosing your deeper intimate needs. Bring romance back into your life by becoming sensitive to your partner's needs and desires. Decide this is what you want and do whatever it takes to achieve it with the person you have chosen as your partner for life.

> **Respect, admiration and love are all earned. Trust and honesty are essential fundamentals**

Loving, long-lasting relationships

We posed the question and asked many people to answer **what does it take to have a loving, long-lasting relationship?** We wonder what your reply would be? Here are some of the replies we received:

- 'Be generous in all things' MALE, MID FIFTIES.
- 'The looser the rein, the tighter the hold' FEMALE, EARLY FORTIES.
- 'Have patience, love, commitment and long-term common goals' MALE, LATE TWENTIES.
- 'Compromise, common sense, consideration and patience' FEMALE, MID THIRTIES.

- 'Loyalty' FEMALE, EARLY FIFTIES.
- 'Communication and compatability' MALE, LATE FORTIES.
- 'Maintain the gifts which were so important when we were children: touching and sensuality' FEMALE, EARLY FORTIES.
- 'Common goals, romance and being able to cope with the changes in the relationship' MALE, MID THIRTIES.
- 'Both having patience, tolerance and being able to listen and communicate with each other' FEMALE, MID FIFTIES.
- 'Mutual respect for each other and understanding that each party may have other interests; for example, sporting, career etc. outside the relationship' MALE, EARLY FIFTIES.
- 'Consideration for your partner's feelings and needs. Trust is important too, and by this I mean you need to show you can be trusted and are responsible. Earn the trust before expecting them to trust you. Having open communication, being cooperative and flexible are very important, but above all else, it is important to have fun and laughter' FEMALE, MID TWENTIES.
- 'Understanding on both sides' FEMALE, EARLY FORTIES.
- 'It takes a great deal of trust and tolerance from both sides. In a relationship you must take the good with the bad. Most important, you should be the best of friends' FEMALE, EARLY THIRTIES.
- 'Be sensual' FEMALE, LATE FORTIES.
- 'It takes a sense of humour, time made to spend together, doing things you enjoy and lots of talking time' FEMALE, MID FORTIES.
- 'Relationships are like riding a bumpy road. You either have to see the potholes and go around them, or experience the shake up along the way. To be successful there must be a constant awareness of the other person. You must talk about

your grievances and come to a peaceful understanding' FEMALE, EARLY SIXTIES.
- 'Get the problems out in the open. Be emotionally honest with each other' MALE, LATE THIRTIES.
- 'Be open-minded, flexible and have an element of adventure in the relationship' FEMALE, LATE FORTIES.
- 'If you want to risk having a fling with someone else, weigh up whether what you are gaining is better than what you are losing' FEMALE, EARLY FORTIES.
- 'It's acting and speaking to each other in a loving way; having empathy with your mate and being supportive no matter what. And cutting out the sarcasm! It's important to act as a team and do things together, and probably most of all keep your sense of humour. As an afterthought, a little sex here and there helps too' MALE, EARLY EIGHTIES.

A thought to inspire you on your journey: 'man cannot discover new oceans, until he has courage to lose sight of the shore'.

If you have been becalmed too long, reassess your direction and invite your partner in love to enjoy the adventure with you. We salute your courage, your sensuality, your relationships and your life. May your journey be colourful, romantic, sensual and seductive.

Recommended reading

Babbitt, Edwin, *The Principles of Light and Colour*, Citadel Press, Secauscus, NJ, 1967.

Birren, Faber, *Colour Psychology and Colour Therapy*, Citadel Press, Secauscus, NJ, 1980.

Godek, G., *1001 Ways to be Romantic*, Margaret Gee Publishing, Sydney, 1991.

Lennon, Robin, *Home Design from the Inside Out*, Penguin, New York, 1997.

Luscher, Max, *The Luscher Color Test*, Random House, New York, 1969.

Malandro, L.A. & Barker, L., *Nonverbal Communication*, Addison Wesley, USA, 1983.

Morris, Desmond, *The Human Animal*, BBC Books, London, 1994.

Sharpe, Deborah, *The Psychology of Colour and Design*, Nelson-Hall, Chicago, 1974.

Steffert, Beverley, *The Rhythms of Love*, HarperCollins, London, 1992.

Tannen, Deborah, *You Just Don't Understand*, Random House, Sydney, 1990.